T0323505

Cultural Safety in Aotearoa New Zealand

Second edition

In this second edition of *Cultural Safety in Aotearoa New Zealand*, editor Dianne Wepa presents a range of theoretical and practice-based perspectives adopted by experienced educators who are active in cultural safety education. Thoroughly revised to incorporate the latest methods and research, this edition reflects updates in government policies and nursing practices, and features new chapters on ethical considerations when working cross-culturally, as well as the legislative requirements of the Nursing Council of New Zealand.

Each chapter includes key terms and concepts, practice examples providing content from healthcare workers' everyday experiences, reflective questions to encourage the assimilation of ideas into practice, and references to allow further exploration of the issues discussed.

Cultural Safety in Aotearoa New Zealand will equip students, tutors, managers, policy analysts and others involved in the delivery of health care with the tools to acknowledge the importance of cultural difference in achieving health and well-being in diverse communities.

Dianne Wepa is an Associate Lecturer at the Auckland University of Technology, New Zealand, and at the time of publication was completing her PhD in Māori health.

Cultural Safety in Aotearoa New Zealand

Edited by Dianne Wepa

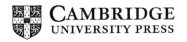

CAMBRIDGE
UNIVERSITY PRESS

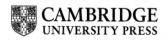

Shaftesbury Road, Cambridge CB2 8EA, United Kingdom

One Liberty Plaza, 20th Floor, New York, NY 10006, USA

477 Williamstown Road, Port Melbourne, VIC 3207, Australia

314–321, 3rd Floor, Plot 3, Splendor Forum, Jasola District Centre, New Delhi – 110025, India

103 Penang Road, #05–06/07, Visioncrest Commercial, Singapore 238467

Cambridge University Press is part of Cambridge University Press & Assessment, a department of the University of Cambridge.

We share the University's mission to contribute to society through the pursuit of education, learning and research at the highest international levels of excellence.

www.cambridge.org
Information on this title: www.cambridge.org/9781107477445

© Cambridge University Press & Assessment 2015

First published by Pearson in 2004
Second edition published by Cambridge University Press & Assessment 2015 (version 7, June 2021)
Cover designed by Marianna Berek-Lewis

A catalogue record for this publication is available from the British Library

A Cataloguing-in-Publication entry is available from the catalogue of the National Library of Australia at www.nla.gov.au

ISBN   978-1-107-47744-5   Paperback

....

Every effort has been made in preparing this book to provide accurate and up-to-date information which is in accord with accepted standards and practice at the time of publication. Although case histories are drawn from actual cases, every effort has been made to disguise the identities of the individuals involved. Nevertheless, the authors, editors and publishers can make no warranties that the information contained herein is totally free from error, not least because clinical standards are constantly changing through research and regulation. The authors, editors and publishers therefore disclaim all liability for direct or consequential damages resulting from the use of material contained in this book. Readers are strongly advised to pay careful attention to information provided by the manufacturer of any drugs or equipment that they plan to use.

Foreword

The 1980s was a transformative decade, both in a positive and negative sense. The reforming Labour Government (1984–1989) dismantled the contract that had existed from the 1930s and which had underpinned community and national welfare. But simultaneously, they also recognised Māori as tangata whenua in new ways and restored the Treaty of Waitangi as the (partial) basis of law and policy.

In this environment, how professional communities understood their own practice, the effects of that practice on client communities and the relationship with Māori came in for new scrutiny. Nursing was to take a particular step in the late 1980s, which was to prove especially significant.

Irihapeti Ramsden was to be involved in a series of hui in the late 1980s from which emerged the notion of cultural safety. Her secondment to the Department of Education in 1988 and her authorship of *Kawa Whakaruruhau* in 1990 helped develop and refine the concept and to implement it in nursing education. Along with Karl Pulotu-Endermann, I worked alongside Irihapeti in a number of nursing programmes to develop the content and principles of cultural safety as did other nursing educators. Irihapeti was a force to be reckoned with and she developed a particular approach that required an understanding of a colonial history, a sense of how culture affects individuals and professional practice, and what principles were relevant to nursing practice. In all of this, Irihapeti was clear that, while Māori should be beneficiaries of cultural safety, kawa whakaruruhau was to apply to any situation where the nurse and patient were of a different ethnicity. Her chapter in this book conveys something of her role and vision as one of the pioneers in transforming nursing education.

There was significant opposition and criticism to cultural safety in the early 1990s from some nursing students and lecturers, and in the wider community. The Nursing Council of New Zealand chose to initiate a review and invited Erihapeti Murchison and myself to visit and consider how cultural safety was being taught in all 16 polytechnics. Our experience was that competency and implementation varied, and our finding was that, while flawed in some respects, cultural safety was critical to contemporary nursing and ought to be retained. But we recommended that resourcing and how cultural safety was being taught needed to be improved. Erihapeti took the view that some aspects (cf. marae visits) should not be compulsory because this did not send the right message;

that a basic respect for other cultures was as important as any educational principle; and that if cultural safety was to succeed in its aims, then it needed more commitment from nursing educators and providers, and from the wider health community.

This book contributes to an understanding of why cultural safety is important to nursing in contemporary New Zealand. As far as I am concerned, the adoption and development of kawa whakaruruhau/cultural safety has been one of the most significant developments in modern nursing practice, made ever more important by the growing ethnic diversity of New Zealand communities and the centrality of Māori as tangata whenua. It has been an innovative step in providing a new paradigm, not only in relation to nursing education, but also with respect to how nursing is practised in Aotearoa New Zealand.

Kia Kaha.

Distinguished Professor Paul Spoonley FRSNZ
Pro Vice-Chancellor
College of Humanities and Social Sciences
Massey University
New Zealand

Contents

Contributors

About the editor

Dianne is of Ngāti Kahungunu descent. She has a background in mental health social work, clinical/cultural supervision and nursing education. As an associate lecturer at Auckland University of Technology, Dianne has developed expert knowledge in the field of cultural safety education and Māori health. She has presented at conferences throughout New Zealand, the South Pacific, the United States and Canada. She has published textbooks and journal articles in cultural safety and clinical supervision. Currently, Dianne is studying towards completing her PhD in health with a focus on patient safety within the hospital and community settings in Hawke's Bay.

About the authors

Liz Banks is a nurse advisor at the Nursing Council of New Zealand, New Zealand.

Ruth Crawford is Principal Lecturer in the School of Nursing at the Eastern Institute of Technology, New Zealand.

Ruth De Souza is Director of Community Engagement and Coordinator of the Bachelor of Nursing (Community Health) at Monash University, Australia.

Isabel Dyck is Professor Emeritus in the School of Geography at Queen Mary College, University of London, United Kingdom.

Sallie Greenwood is the Principal Academic Staff Member for the Centre for Health and Social Practice at the Waikato Institute of Technology, New Zealand.

Riripeti Haretuku is the Managing Director of Mauriora Associates Limited, New Zealand.

Huhana Hickey is a research fellow in the Taupua Waiora Centre for Māori Health Research at the Auckland University of Technology, New Zealand.

Robin Kearns is Professor of Geography in the School of Environment at the University of Auckland, New Zealand.

Maureen Kelly is the Education and Standards Manager at the Nursing Council of New Zealand, New Zealand.

Ngaire Kerse is Head of School of Population Health and Professor of General Practice and Primary Health Care at the University of Auckland, New Zealand.

Liz Kiata is a research fellow in the Faculty of Health at the Queensland University of Technology, Australia.

Rosemary McEldowney is Head of the School of Health at Charles Darwin University, Australia.

Elaine Papps is a senior lecturer in the School of Nursing at the Eastern Institute of Technology, New Zealand.

Thelma Puckey is a registered comprehensive nurse working for the Community Mental Health Services, Toowoomba, Queensland, Australia.

Irihapeti Ramsden belonged to the people of Ngai Tahupōtiki and Ranitane. She was a Māori nurse educator, and conducted seminars on cultural safety, the Treaty of Waitangi and Māori health issues. In 2003 she was invested as an Officer of the New Zealand Order of Merit.

Fran Richardson is a lecturer in the School of Health at Charles Darwin University, Australia.

Deb Spence is a senior lecturer in the Faculty of Health and Environmental Sciences at the Auckland University of Technology, New Zealand.

Katarina Jean Te Huia, of Ngāti Kahungunu descent, is a midwife, lactation consultant and sexual health practitioner, and Director of Midwifery Choices Limited, Havelock North, New Zealand.

Rachael Vernon is Associate Professor and Associate Head of School in the School of Nursing and Midwifery at the University of South Australia, Australia.

Denise Wilson is the Professor of Māori Health in the Centre for Māori Health Research, Faculty of Health and Environmental Studies at the Auckland University of Technology, New Zealand.

Introduction

Kia ora and welcome to the second edition of *Cultural Safety in Aotearoa New Zealand*. It has been almost 20 years since cultural safety education became an integral part of the nursing and midwifery curriculum. A testament to the longevity of cultural safety has been its ability to remain relevant within the 21st century. Such relevance has culminated into the Nursing Council of New Zealand's (2011) *Guidelines for Cultural Safety, the Treaty of Waitangi and Māori Health in Nursing Education and Practice*.

This edition builds on the first edition of *Cultural Safety in Aotearoa New Zealand* whereby chapters have been reviewed due to feedback from the health and education sector. The end result has been the inclusion of chapters focused on whānau-centred practice, disability and competence. Chapter 2, written by professionals from the Nursing Council of New Zealand ('the Nursing Council') on competencies required for registered nurses' scope of practice, is of significance within this second edition. Direct passages from the Nursing Council's competencies are linked to real-life experiences so that students can become familiar with such requirements at an earlier stage within their respective programmes.

As with the first edition, the first three chapters set the scene with a discussion on the concepts within cultural safety and historical events that led to its inclusion by schools of nursing and midwifery. The foundations of cultural safety follow with six chapters focusing on concepts around culture, ethnicity, the Treaty of Waitangi, prejudice, ethics and research. The next eight chapters focus on fields of practice where practitioners have contributed their views on child/youth/family, mental health, midwifery, minority cultures, the aged, gender, Māori health initiatives and disability. I sincerely hope that this text will be useful for classroom and practice-based teaching and I welcome any feedback to improve the learning experience for students and health outcomes for all recipients of care in Aotearoa New Zealand.

Dianne Wepa

A note on the cover image

The manu tukutuku claims tino rangatiratanga and all that is involved in responsibility, governance, protection and relationship. The kākahu with broad tāniko band is based on the kaitaka cloak – a garment of mana of the highest prestige – something for all health professionals to be attuned to in their care of persons and the tapu of the body. The gold and silver leaf at the base talks about the sacred tie between humanity and land – the physical/whenua and the spiritual/waiora.

The tāniko on the kaitaka has been worked to talk about awareness; colours around the kaitaka and manu aute are healing/good health colours.

Gabrielle Belz

part 1

Setting the scene

1 Towards cultural safety

Irihapeti Ramsden

Learning objectives

Having studied this chapter, you will be able to:

- be familiar with the name of two models of Māori health;

- be able to describe the connection between colonisation, the Treaty of Waitangi and Māori health;

- understand the difference between nursing someone regardless of their uniqueness and being regardful of their difference;

- be able to critique the notion of multiculturalism within nursing;

- be able to describe cultural differences beyond ethnicity;

- be able to understand the origin of the term cultural safety;

- describe the importance of each of the following:
  - › nurses' attitudes towards patients
  - › recognition and understanding of the powerlessness of patients
  - › the centrality of open-mindedness and self-awareness.

Key terms and concepts

- colonisation

- culturally safe health professional

- model for negotiated and equal partnership

- multiculturalism

- power of nurses

- Te wheke

- the Treaty of Waitangi

- Whare Tapa Whā

Introduction

This chapter explores the historical relationship between the health status of Māori, the Treaty of Waitangi and health services in Aotearoa New Zealand at the time when cultural safety developed. The clarification of these issues was necessary to enable me to work effectively in the teaching environment and introduce what was essentially new and revolutionary material to nursing and midwifery students. A chronological overview to the evolution of cultural safety following the immediate period after my initial teaching experiences in 1988 through to 2001 is presented. I wish to convey to the reader some essence of the sheer speed, over this thirteen-year period, at which cultural safety development has taken place within New Zealand nursing and midwifery professions.

Practice examples are given to assist the reader to recognise and understand the powerlessness of patients and the power of nurses.

Historical analysis

The effects of colonisation and the growing awareness through the 1970s and 1980s of the ongoing and long-term impact of the colonisation process on Māori health outcomes were a critical impetus for the development of cultural safety. As political awareness and activity among Māori during this time began to increase, gatherings of Māori people working in education, welfare and justice, and health were also meeting together, many for the first time, to discuss those areas of concern in relation to Māori.

The attention of health authorities to the state of Māori health had been reinforced by the participants of a hui held at Hoani Waititi Marae Auckland, in March 1984. Primary Māori concerns had formerly been land, education and welfare. Now the attention turned to health. This well-attended gathering of Māori health professionals was the first national hui to be held on Māori health and was a focus for a large number of concerns, including the need for research, the requirement that Māori should be involved in Māori health service design and delivery, and the need for government to recognise the growing body of evidence that Māori health and disease issues were different from those of the general population.

Durie (1994) states that there were hui throughout the country in the early part of the decade which accepted a model of health incorporating taha wairua (spiritual health), taha hinengaro (mental health), taha tinana (physical health) and taha whānau (family health), and that this became widely accepted as the preferred Māori definition of health. Hui Whakaoranga also recommended that health and education institutions recognise culture as a positive resource. Spiritual and emotional factors as contributors to health and well-being were emphasised at the hui. Although Durie admits that the Whare Tapa Whā model is simple, 'even simplistic', it had immediate appeal for Māori and Pākehā alike. For example, the model was adopted widely by nursing schools and formed the basis for the philosophy of the inaugural curriculum of the Waiariki Polytechnic Nursing School at Rotorua which was set up in 1985. A further model appeared during this period which has enjoyed a level of acceptance, Te Wheke (Pere, 1991), which represents the tentacles of an octopus, each concerned with an aspect of health or illness or community and family.

The Treaty of Waitangi

The formal agreement between Māori hapū and the British Crown took the form of a treaty written in both Māori and English which was signed initially at Waitangi in the Bay of Islands in 1840. Later versions were signed at several other sites around the country.

Although the first article in Māori ultimately accommodated a very loosely worded transfer of sovereignty, the Treaty of Waitangi made significant guarantees of Crown protection of Māori taonga/treasures while guaranteeing that Māori also retained control over Māori resources in Article Two. In Article Three, the Treaty guaranteed Māori the same rights and privileges as British subjects enjoyed in 1840. In common with all treaties, this one was written with the future in mind. Although the Treaty was declared a simple nullity in 1877, because it had never been incorporated into New Zealand law by a specific Act of Parliament, it was acknowledged as the founding document of New Zealand in 1992 (Durie, 1994).

Contact with introduced diseases, war and poverty contributed to a dramatic reduction in the Māori population from 1769 to 1890. The Māori population, although inaccurately measured, was clearly in continuous decline. Mason Durie states that the Māori population had dropped by a third in less than a century and quoted a prophecy from 1884 in *Whaiora*:

> Just as the Norwegian rat has displaced the Māori rat, as introduced plants have displaced Māori plants so the white man will replace the Māori. (Durie, 1994, p. 32)

Fortunately this prophecy was not fulfilled but the Māori population remained essentially rurally based until after 1945, when the migration to cities accelerated. As most of the non-Māori population was already urban based there was little real contact between Māori and non-Māori until the mid-1970s when Māori began to recover numbers, and make a critical impact on the social climate of New Zealand.

There has been much debate and speculation over the contemporary relevance of the Treaty to health care and the application of the words of the Treaty as agreed to in 1840. Debate has also been consistent over the meanings and interpretation of the differing texts in Māori and in English. Fiduciary obligations, although unwritten, are understood to mean that both parties must act in good faith toward each other.

The practice has emerged of extracting and addressing principles of the Treaty rather than attempting to analyse and understand the exact intention of every word in the English and the Māori texts. Although Durie states that extracting principles and applying them to contemporary health situations has its limitations, the practice has acquired popularity in assisting people to translate the Treaty guarantees into possibilities for action (Durie, 1989). There is a range of principles which have been developed over time by different organisations but the ones which have acquired the most currency in daily society are the three which were produced by the Royal Commission on Social Policy (1988). They are the principles of partnership, participation and protection. The ideas behind these principles have been variously interpreted according to the organisation which has employed them.

Graphic evidence of the status of the health of Māori people was recorded in a report to the Minister of Māori Affairs called *Progress Towards Closing Social and Economic Gaps between Māori and Non-Māori* (Te Puni Kokiri, 2000). Comparison with non-Māori as demonstrated in this report upholds the argument of many Māori that since the Crown took over the management of Māori health and disease status, Māori have been consistently failed by all Crown agencies concerned with health service and delivery to the indigenous people of New Zealand.

Since the Treaty of Waitangi Act 1975, the Treaty has grown steadily in the public attention. Pushed largely by Māori urban activism to address the social and economic consequences of legislatively induced poverty (Durie, 1994), the establishment of the Waitangi Tribunal was seen as a significant outlet for Māori frustrations. Publicity given to the succession of cases and the landmark decisions that it made in respect of tribal claims against the

Crown enabled Treaty issues to assume an importance which they had not had over the previous 100 years. The Treaty became a focus for race relations activity, particularly in respect to property rights. Māori attempts to assert their arguments regarding these matters often caused vituperative comment from all levels of New Zealand society, ranging from radio talkback to the 1975 Court of Appeal decisions on the role and function of the Waitangi Tribunal.

Political issues in relation to the Treaty of Waitangi or health and economic disparity were unexplored in nursing education and evolving approaches to matters relating to the health of the indigenous people were happening from a 'biculturalist or multiculturalist' angle in which the primary emphasis is on ethnicity and exotic cultural difference. All exotic or outside groups of people came to be included in the multicultural paradigm.

In New Zealand the term *biculturalism* came to represent the relationship between Māori and others, particularly the Crown. This gave rise to a constant argument that other cultures were not being given adequate consideration in any or all contexts in which Māori were contesting for resources or arguing for attention to Māori-defined political issues. The impression was given that Māori were activating simply for their own purposes and that other cultures needed patronising and defending. The idea that there were intact groups of people which could be called cultures was considered to be common sense and normal and was referred to in everyday conversation as though cultures were measurable and easily definable.

Many Māori have identified health as a major issue worthy of a case to be taken before the Waitangi Tribunal. Although such a case has not yet been constructed there is continuous discussion of the possibility of doing so in Māori circles. Māori nurses have been involved in a case against the Crown in respect to Māori health (Waitangi Tribunal, personal communication, Wellington, 2000). Because the New Zealand public, including most Māori, had so little knowledge of the Treaty, its content and its future implications, the response of the public was volatile and usually ad hoc. Loud protest erupted against Māori activism or non-Māori support for Māori activism, on the radio, in the bias of television and newspaper reporting and letters to the Editors. Cartoons which drew on negative Māori stereotypes and other media further enhanced a climate of vitriolic and angry attitudes and behaviour toward Māori attempts to make change.

Terms which applied to the study of issues of Māori health and disease varied at this period but the most commonly employed were: *biculturalism, cultural differences, cultural awareness,* and *cultural sensitivity*. None of these terms addressed the political context in which Māori ill health was happening. The political link between the Treaty and its guarantees of equity including the possibility of equal health status with other New Zealanders in Article Three had not been correlated in the teaching of nurses. The discussion of issues of power and Māori representation in the health service lay in the very near future. It was in this climate that I first encountered classes of nursing students.

Learning and teaching: students as teachers

Although I had an undergraduate university degree which was unusual for a nurse practitioner or a nursing teacher in 1986, I had no theoretical training in teaching, let alone teaching in the delicate area of antiracism or attitude formation and change. I had little formal analysis of the situations around me and no classroom experience. I entered the teaching environment with few tools other than my own nursing education and practice and a deep commitment to help create positive change.

The following year, the Standing Committee on Māori Health (1987) recommended that the Treaty of Waitangi be regarded as a foundation for good health. I was beginning my teaching practice at a very interesting time in New Zealand history. Although my first attempt to include Māori health issues in the curriculum of the Parumoana Polytechnic, a 35-hour paper called 'Intercultural Nursing' was the subject of congratulations in a letter from the Nursing Council of New Zealand, there was no formal agreement between the Council as a professional body set up under statute, and Māori, based on the Treaty of Waitangi.

The idea of a cultural checklist in which heavily stereotyped *cultures* were able to be predicted by nurses leading to insight on the part of the nurse and conformity and compliance on the part of the patient (Bruni, 1988), was something which I later came to describe as a cultural smorgasbord (Ramsden, 2000). The metaphor was one of 'cultural tourism' or 'voyeurism', where the nurse stood outside, secure in the culture of nursing, and surveyed the patient from the viewpoint of their interesting exoticism. The interesting exoticism was usually in deficit compared with the culture of nursing and allowed the nurse to be patronising and powerful. There were no grounds for the nurse to consider that change in their own attitude and self-knowledge was needed before any trust could be established.

It was also assumed that nurses could speak for the perceived needs of people from other ethnic groups. The popular concept of culture remained ethnicity-based while groups of people with clearly defined commonalities, sharing kinship, world views and ways of existing in the world – such as religious groups, for example Jehovah's Witnesses, closed religious sects, or the Salvation Army – were not seen as exotic cultures. Nor did nurses see themselves as having the right to investigate or provide commentary on groups of people in the way that they felt they could about Māori.

A further philosophical underpinning of the multicultural debate, and relevant to the nursing and midwifery education context, arose when Māori tried to assert political status as First Peoples. The disagreement lay in the nursing notion that all people should be nursed equally regardless of their difference from nurses or from each other. This ideology was expressed by the National Action Group in The Aims and Scope of Nursing (1988) that saw nurses as being providers of care irrespective of differences such as nationality, culture, creed, colour, sex, political or religious belief or social status. Very similar words are reiterated in the International Council of Nurses' Code for Nurses which states:

> The need for nursing is universal. Inherent in nursing is respect for life, dignity, and rights of man (sic). It is unrestricted by considerations of nationality, race, creed, colour, age, sex, politics or social status. (Johnstone and Ecker, 2001, p. 403)

The report which I wrote in 1990, *Kawa Whakaruruhau: Cultural Safety in Nursing Education in Aotearoa* (Ramsden, 1990), refuted the premise that people could be nursed regardless of all the elements which made them unique in the world. In the introduction I wrote:

> The idea of the nurse ignoring the way in which people measure and define their humanity is unrealistic and inappropriate . . . People are still prepared to die in order to maintain their cultural, religious and territorial integrity. It is not the place of the nursing service to attempt to deny the vital differences between people, however altruistic the rationale may be. (Ramsden, 1990, p. 1)

In the graduation speech to the Diploma of Nursing students at Nelson Polytechnic, I wrote that:

> Only one word needs to be altered in order to suitably change the old nursing philosophy to become appropriate for the end of the 20th century and onward

into the 21st. That word is *irrespective* . . . Nurses must become respective of the nationality of human beings, the culture of human beings, the age, the sex the political and the religious beliefs of other members of the human race. (Ramsden, 1988)

These statements lay two years into the future. Initially, I too adopted the multiculturalist/ethnic approach. Although I was uncomfortable about it from the beginning of my teaching experience I was not clear about how to analyse or express my diffidence. Fuimaono Karl Puloto Endemann, then Deputy Head of School Palmerston North Polytechnic School of Nursing, commented passionately on multiculturalism in his interview for this project:

I hate multiculturalism . . . yes I do . . . I hate it. Hate to me is a very powerful word. Because what multiculturalism does, it actually demeans people. I always say that for us Pacific Islanders it makes us into the hula girls, and the chop suey and rice kind of sentiment, like that's what we are right across the board . . . If we are all the same, how come you are rich and I'm not? (Karl Puloto-Endemann, interviewee)

The ideology of multiculturalism was deeply held by students and was expressed by many of them in a microcosm of New Zealand society. Common statements were:

- 'We are all the same in New Zealand.'
- 'What is different about Māoris?'
- 'Why should they have more than us?'
- 'We are all one people. I grew up/went to school with Māoris and they were the same as we were.'
- 'Māoris have special privileges that we don't such as scholarships.'
- 'New Zealand is a multicultural society, what about all the other cultures?'

I realised that it was essential to place this kind of discourse into a social context and then somehow teach what I had found to nursing students (Wetherell and Potter, 1992). From the beginning I tried to introduce an analysis of racism in New Zealand communities and describe its effect on Māori people. I began by describing differences between Polynesian and United Kingdom-based cultures indulging myself, in a naive way, in stereotypes of each group. The cultural checklist approach was satisfying for most students because it gave them something to quantify and to repeat back in assignments. For a short while I found it more convenient to teach from this position but my own life experience imposed itself on the information I was dispensing. It was clear that cultural stereotypes were simplistic and untrue and that the complexity of post-colonial cause and effects on New Zealand society must be taught. I came to struggle hard against the checklist mentality and consequently made my own work much harder. Later I became able to use the Treaty as a teaching framework but as yet there was no backup from the statuary nursing institution which could help teachers to formulate and uphold such a framework.

In 1994 the Nursing Council of New Zealand, the statuary regulatory body for nurses and midwives, acknowledged the Treaty of Waitangi in a three-year strategic plan (Nursing Council of New Zealand, 1994). Part of this plan identified the role of the Council in relation to the Treaty of Waitangi as a critical strategic issue. As a Crown agent, the Nursing Council is morally bound to observe the principles of the Treaty of Waitangi, as are all Crown agencies although the Treaty of Waitangi does not appear in the Nurses Act 1977.

> The Nursing Council of New Zealand is in effect, an agent of the Crown through its statutory role in the maintenance of standards of education and practice for nurses and midwives. It is empowered by the Nurses Act 1977 to act as such an agent by setting and monitoring standards to ensure safe and competent care for the public of New Zealand. (Papps, 2002, p. 98)

In an environment of assimilation and denial of difference, this was the worst place to start teaching. Students were largely from the New Zealand islands and descended from United Kingdom immigrants. They were mostly young female school leavers with little travel or cross-cultural experience. The polytechnic was situated in a low socio-economic area. Although the ratio of people from Pacific Island communities was much higher in Porirua than other parts of Wellington, anecdotally, intimate interaction between groups was low apart from public activities such as attendance at schools.

These young people had come to be nurses and the work on racism, cultures and difference that I was offering appeared to have little bearing on nursing which was a profession in their view which cared for people regardless of who they were. Students were very clear about expressing their opinions. If they did not see the relevance of what I was teaching they protested loudly, ignored my presentations, spoke during visiting speakers' presentations and eventually boycotted my classes. At one point I had only three students attending class; one was an older Samoan woman, another a scholarship student from the Solomon Islands and the third, a Pākehā who had arranged her hair into three stiffly pointed projections dyed bright green. These three students stayed with me all year and I am grateful to them for their gentleness and patience to this day.

What I did learn from the students' challenges?

Like me, the students lacked the capacity to analyse what was happening to them in my classes. They had less knowledge of the Treaty of Waitangi than I did and they were confronted and affronted by my challenges to their lifetime beliefs about race relations in New Zealand. Patti Lather (1991), in discussing the development of emancipatory social theory, is clear that an empirical stance is required which is open ended and grounded in respect for human capacity but also needs to be profoundly sceptical of appearances and *'common sense'* (Lather, 1991, p. 65).

While I was learning to explain issues in a professional context it was not done quickly enough to meet the students' immediate educational and emotional needs, and their responses became collective and punitive. They exercised what power they could by refusing to participate in my classes as much as possible and I exercised what power I could by presenting them with information which I thought important for their practice. It was also critical that I did not demonstrate the passion I felt for this topic; although it was permissible for me to show stimulation, excitement and enthusiasm in the teaching of my other subject, surgical nursing.

Systems of education are not neutral (Freire, 1996) and are established to meet a set of agendas. Roy Shuker (1987, p. 21) argues that the schooling system functions as a state construction to reproduce labour power and the means of production:

> This involves producing a labour force with ideas, values and practices which are consistent with, and in acceptance of existing power relations.

There was little question that the students who were entering nursing courses and had been educated in New Zealand (the majority) were fixed in their views on race relations and the locus of power. The power clearly lay with Anglo-derived middle to upper middle class members of New Zealand society and not with Māori or other marginalised groups of people.

I learned that unless I could show an effect in the environment of health and disease, then teaching the cause, i.e. land deprivation, social injustice and/or racism, was almost pointless. This was material students had never been exposed to. It was critical that like any other historical facts they made sense to the student and should be presented in the correct framework of their education. I needed to ask myself, why were they in the course? Then I had to address the facts that I was wishing to teach to the reason for the presence of students, which was to become graduate nurses and to deliver excellent service.

The next part of my developing pedagogy was to relate the facts to nursing practice. Here my nursing practice in the Porirua community stood me in good stead. I was able to illustrate the relationship of history to the people and communities around us and to the disparities and facts of life with which most of the students were more than familiar. It was also possible to link the Treaty of Waitangi breaches to health and social disparity. When I began to draw on practice my classes refilled and I was able to learn as I went along with students. Although we were learning different facts, we were both learning about power, mine to create emancipatory change in students' view of the world and students to create teaching which would match their needs to become nursing professionals. Since I was also working with students in clinical practice, it became possible to translate classroom teaching to the hospital or community environments and again back to the classroom. The following three practice examples illustrate particular aspects of this.

Practice examples

The importance of attitude, recognising and understanding the powerlessness of patients and the power of nurses, and the centrality of open-mindedness and self-awareness, are illustrated in the following practice examples.

Attitudes matter

Practice example 1

Attitudes matter and when people need a nurse or need health care they are in a vulnerable state, extremely vulnerable, and they need respect and they need to be treated with love and justice.
(Isabelle Sherrard, interviewee)

A Māori woman was admitted to a local hospital seriously ill from a rupture of a hydatid cyst in her abdomen. She was deeply unconscious when the student nurse and I came to help with her care in the Intensive Care Unit. We joined the ward round and were present during a full staff meeting around her bed as she lay unconscious, her breathing maintained by a respirator. Apart from her present condition the woman did not look as though she had been healthy or prosperous prior to admission. She was tired looking, had no teeth and was clinically obese, white roots were growing through her hair. Although comment was made only on her obesity it was clear by the attitude that staff did not consider this woman to have been compliant when first diagnosed and that she had presented an extreme surgical risk. There was general conversation about her non-compliance with attendance at clinics and her irresponsible attitude toward her condition. The atmosphere during the discussion between surgeons was that she had brought a great deal of her trouble upon herself by not turning up at clinics and disappearing from the surgeons' supervision until the dramatic rupture of the cyst.

It was clear that the student nurse was listening to the conversation carefully and that she was also absorbing the non-verbal communication that was happening between the lines. We decided to do some investigation into the background of this unfortunate woman. As we went carefully through her notes we discovered that she was a sole caregiver of eight children, some of whom were pre-school grandchildren. She had been trying to keep her family together by working a little piece of land with sheep and share milking, hence the exposure to the possibility of hydatids. The pressures of child rearing, poverty and prioritising for the needs of others had caused her to forgo her trips to town to attend at the hospital. There was one phone call of apology for inability to attend the clinic in the notes.

When the student had put together the background to the situation this woman was in, I asked her to present her findings to the class, including the unspoken communication. The student nurse made an excellent and clearly thought out analysis of what she had seen and heard, as well as not heard but had understood, and she unknowingly gave me two of the objectives that I later brought to cultural safety. They were:

> to educate student nurses and midwives not to blame the victims of historical process for their current plights;

> to educate student nurses and midwives to examine their own realities and the attitudes they bring to each new person they encounter in their practice.

Recognising powerlessness and power

Practice example 2

A student and I were working together in a busy surgical ward. A young man was admitted from Western Samoa for elective surgery for an inguinal hernia. The young man spoke very hesitant English and preferred to sit quietly cross-legged on his bed waiting for something to happen. The student and I were anxious that there was no interpreter to assist with the preparation for surgery and as the time for his premedication approached it became obvious that nobody had spoken with this young man or helped him with his preparation. He still required a pubic shave, skin preparation and theatre garb. Finally we went to the nurse who was caring for him and asked about his preparation and suggested that an interpreter would be helpful – she told us to find one for him. Finally, as the time for theatre approached,

we found a young Samoan nurse from another ward, negotiated her release from her ward and got to the bed just as the nurse arrived to shave the patient, the nurse with the intramuscular pre-medication hove into view and the theatre trolley arrived. The patient became frustrated as the interpreter tried to explain the procedures and each health worker pushed to complete their tasks. The patient was insulted by the attempts of the female nurse to shave his groin, something unacceptable in his own cultural environment, the staff were also frustrated as time passed.

This confusion had clearly arisen because of a poor initial nursing assessment and resultant inadequate planning on the part of the primary care nurse and the patient did his very best in a foreign setting to cope with the nursing mismanagement that had been visited upon him. Had the patient responded in ways that the staff considered inappropriate, for example by shouting or physically resisting attempts to touch him, the possibility of his being blamed for behaving in ways which were upsetting to staff and ward routines would have been very high. Intervention by the interpreter, who fortunately was a nurse (often non-health professionals are informally involved as interpreters) and could explain what was happening, and the locating of a male nurse to do the shave, saved the situation from being potentially quite disruptive to all concerned. The sheer grace and patience of the young man also made it possible for him to negotiate his way through the mosaic of dilemmas.

The students analysed this situation and applied the objectives of cultural safety to it, recognising the powerlessness of the patient and the power of the nurse to create an environment in which these quandaries need not have developed. Had the nurse made an accurate assessment of the patient's language status at admission, most of the confusion could have been avoided. The issue therefore lay with the practice of the nurse rather than the behaviours of the patient.

Open-minded, self-aware

Practice example 3

At the afternoon shift report, the senior nurse giving the overview of the ward commented that a Samoan woman patient had had over twenty visitors who said they were family that morning, most of whom insisted on staying close to the patient. As the nurse gave this information she rolled her eyes, sighed and looked frustrated. She did not say anything pejorative about the patient or the amount of visitors or them being in the way of nursing cares being carried out, but it was clear that this was what she was thinking. Each time she mentioned the patient she non-verbally expressed impatience and gave the impression that the afternoon staff were in for a trying time.

This dilemma is a particularly good one for student group discussion because it highlights the rapid socialisation of student nurses. Most students by Year Two of their degree programme in my experience, agree with the nurse conveying the non-verbal messages relating to 'inappropriately' sized family groups and other visitors upsetting ward routines and other patients. It takes an exceptional student to detect the underlying racism relating to the definition of family, and to see that the nurses on the previous shift should have negotiated their way through this situation with the large kinship group of the patient and should not have left this situation to become the legacy of the afternoon staff. There can be a range of solutions depending on the circumstances, all of which can lead to successful negotiation and mutually beneficial outcomes. From this type of situation, the final two objectives of cultural safety were drawn:

> to educate student nurses and midwives to be open minded and flexible in their attitudes toward people who are different from themselves, to whom they offer and deliver service;

> to produce a workforce of well-educated, self-aware registered nurses and midwives who are culturally safe to practice, as defined by the people they serve.

The issues highlighted by these practice situations and the teaching which was evolving from them produced dilemmas of their own. Questions arose not only in relation to how such material should be taught but also about who should teach it, how it should be assessed, even where and when it should be taught. Because cross-cultural issues in the New Zealand context were perceived to be between Māori and non-Māori, most practice exemplars and test questions were based in this primary New Zealand relationship. Culture was uncompromisingly seen as ethnicity and it remained difficult to present the diversity of notions of culture which my anthropological training had given me.

It was frustrating to see stereotyping questions used which were pejorative, patronising, treated Māori as exotic and did not relate to the ill health or otherwise of Māori people. Above all, they did not test nursing or midwifery practice. As highly diverse, colonised and urbanised people, there was little that Māori had to show apart from the postcard and tourist imagery. This is what appeared to be built upon when teaching and testing nursing assessments.

> In some ways I think it was easier for Pākehā institutions to dump cultural safety on a Māori or a Māori Department and then it could be, as so many Māori things are, marginalised. That, in the first few years of the programme, was my main fear about how it was developing. I don't particularly want nurses to know how to sing waiata, I want them to treat my mother properly if she's unwell. (Moana Jackson, interviewee)

The newly established Māori Studies Departments in polytechnics were called in to provide Māori teachers who were non-nurses, to assist in this process. This served to enhance the Māori Studies view of Māori health and to entrench it in the systems of teaching nurses and midwives. Māori Studies teachers were not teaching nursing and midwifery because it was not possible for them to do so. In some schools, students were being taught to recite prayers in Māori and being tested on their capacity to remember the prayers, and in others to sing Māori songs and perform dances. Unfortunately remnants of this period still persist in some Schools of nursing and midwifery.

The political and economic realities of life for many Māori people became subsumed by romantic and sentimentalised colonial constructs (Bell, 1992). There was further debate over the place of teaching Māori issues, and for several years it was thought useful to take students to traditional Māori locations to learn about 'the habits and the customs of the natives' (Ramsden and Spoonley, 1994, p. 163). This was comfortably in line with Transcultural Nursing theory (Leininger, 1991). Although the Nursing Council of New Zealand was clear that this practice, if followed at all, should relate to nursing and midwifery educational aims, it remained popular as a group familiarisation process and an enjoyable class outing (Nursing Council of New Zealand, 1996).

For some groups, the outings were not so enjoyable as politicised Māori began to challenge their audiences in a range of ways. My experience taught me that contentious issues such as race relations in New Zealand should not be raised in the first year of any nursing diploma, or later degree programme, for a range of very cogent reasons. A level of trust had not evolved within the class group by early in the first year (sometimes in the first week) when students were often taken out to marae for the 'Māori experience'. Another reason was that Māori students were placed in very emotionally vulnerable situations when they had often not defined their own identities. Students usually did not possess the social or educational building blocks on which to base such information in relation to nursing. By the second year, students had settled as a group and had some clinical experience to compare with classroom theory. As I began to learn the pedagogy which the students helped to teach me, and was more able to integrate practice exemplars having acquired some educational theory, I found my classes remained well attended.

Appointment to the Department of Education

Late in 1987 I was approached by the Department of Education to consider a secondment to research the health needs of young Māori trainees on government pre-employment schemes. This meant relocation to downtown Wellington and entry into education and research politics. At this time I was also appointed to the Education Committee of the Nursing Council of New Zealand, the first Māori appointment to this significant and powerful committee or to any committee on the Council. Nursing and midwifery education was the obvious place to start the work which became known as cultural safety and the juxtaposition of the appointment to the Education Committee and the opportunity to gain a national overview and national influence through the Departmental secondment were extremely fortuitous.

On completion of the research project and the production of the educational video and poster package that emerged from it, I was further employed by the Department of Education to set up and facilitate a hui which was to be concerned with the recruitment and retention of Māori students in nursing courses.

At this period the Department of Education had a position called Senior Education Officer, Nursing, filled by Ms Janet Davidson (who was interviewed for this project), which had responsibility for the overall educational co-ordination of the fifteen polytechnics providing nursing courses. Such was the concern of the Department of Education to respond to the principles of the Treaty of Waitangi and to get Māori health issues successfully integrated into nursing education, that the position offered to me was especially created. The position was called Education Officer, Nursing and Māori Health, and was one of several which were involved with Māori issues in the tertiary sector.

Looking back, it is possible to see that my time in the Department of Education provided an amazing opportunity to translate my prior experience, concerns and emerging insights as a teacher to conceptual and practical strategies for nursing education at a national level. It also provided opportunity to bring together issues of Māori health and the role and place of nurses within healthcare to make a critical difference.

My role was to help co-ordinate curriculum development and course content in all the polytechnics at a national level. This involved a series of visits over the next two years and resulted in the production of *A Model for Negotiated and Equal Partnership* (Ramsden, 1989a) (presented in Figure 1.1), which was accepted by all polytechnics and implemented regionally according to their own community settings. Relationships between local iwi and nursing schools were critical to the model. A most innovative response was the relationship that the Otago Polytechnic Department of Nursing developed with Ngai Tahu, the local tangata whenua, where the School of Nursing and Ngai Tahu co-own the cultural safety curriculum to this day.

In the years following the writing and introduction of the model, discussions with educators teaching in polytechnics at that time have shown me that they regarded it as revolutionising for their thinking and for their practice. It provided a structure and process for moving forward with this aspect of education. It also provided a basis for arguments for obtaining resources.

A number of nurse educators have shared with me that the model came at a time when they were seeking alternative strategies in nursing education, as they recognised the importance of addressing these issues. However, in some places these educators were lone voices.

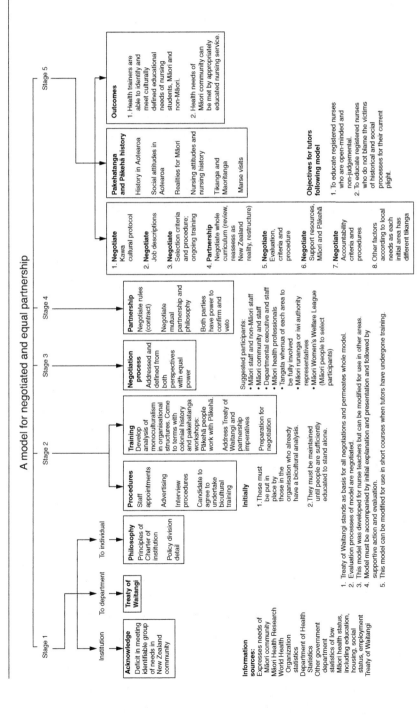

A model for negotiated and equal partnership

A model for negotiated and equal partnership

Stage 1 | Stage 2 | Stage 3 | Stage 4 | Stage 5

Acknowledge
Deficit in meeting identifiable group of needs in New Zealand community

Treaty of Waitangi

Institution — To department — To individual

Philosophy
Principles of Charter of institution

Policy division detail

Procedures
Staff appointments

Advertising

Interview procedures

Candidate to agree to undertake bicultural training

Training
Develop analysis of monoculturalism in organisational structures. Come to terms with colonial history and pakehatanga Pākehā people work with Pākehā.

Address Treaty of Waitangi and partnership imperatives

Preparation for negotiation

Negotiation process
Addressed and defined from both perspectives with equal power

Partnership
Negotiate rules (contract)

Negotiate mutual partnership and philosophy

Both parties have power to confirm and veto

Outcomes
1. Health trainers are able to identify and meet culturally defined educational needs of nursing students, Māori and non-Māori.
2. Health needs of Māori community can be met by appropriately educated nursing service.

Pakehatanga and Pākehā history
History in Aotearoa

Social attitudes in Aotearoa

Realities for Māori

Nursing attitudes and nursing history

Tikanga and Maoritanga

Marae visits

1. **Negotiate**
Kawa cultural protocol
2. **Negotiate**
Job descriptions
3. **Negotiate**
Selection criteria and procedure; ongoing training
4. **Partnership**
Negotiate whole curriculum (review, reassess as New Zealand reality, restructure)
5. **Negotiate**
Evaluation, criteria and procedure
6. **Negotiate**
Support resources, Māori and Pākehā
7. **Negotiate**
Accountability criteria and procedures
8. Other factors according to local needs as each initial area has different tikanga

Objectives for tutors following model
1. To educate registered nurses who are open-minded and non-judgemental.
2. To educate registered nurses who do not blame the victims of historical and social processes for their current plight.

Information sources:
Expresses needs of Māori community

Māori Health Research

World Health Organization statistics

Department of Health Statistics

Other government department statistics of low Māori health status, including education, housing, social status, employment

Treaty of Waitangi

Initially

1. These must be put in place by those in the organisation who already have a bicultural analysis.

2. They must be maintained until people are sufficiently educated to stand alone.

Suggested participants:
- Māori staff and non-Māori staff
- Māori community and staff
- Departmental executive and staff
- Māori health professionals
- Tangata whenua of each area to be fully involved by
- Māori runanga or iwi authority representatives
- Māori Women's Welfare League (Māori people to select participants)

1. Treaty of Waitangi stands as basis for all negotiations and permeates whole model.
2. Evaluation processes of model are negotiated.
3. This model was developed for nurse teachers but can be modified for use in other areas.
4. Model must be accompanied by initial explanation and presentation and followed by supportive action and evaluation.
5. This model can be modified for use in short courses when tutors have undergone training.

FIGURE 1.1 *A model for negotiated and equal partnership*

Hui Waimanawa

The second critical impetus for the development of cultural safety, also associated with my role at this time, was a national hui, the Hui Waimanawa. This hui, which I was commissioned to run in 1988, was significant in several ways. First, the budget allowed me to take the gathering to my home area so that I could be supported in the work by my grandparents and other family who came and sat with me for the week. My grandfather named the gathering, Hui Waimanawa, in recognition of the tears which had been shed over the years of colonisation and to recognise the importance of the hui being able to happen.

Second, since the gathering was concerned with the experience of Māori students, I invited Māori students to take part in the hui which had over a hundred participants. Third, the participation of Māori students produced the term *cultural safety*.

Fourth, the report of the hui and *A Model For Negotiated and Equal Partnership* (Ramsden, 1989a) became critical turning points in the implementation of *cultural safety* into nursing education because they were accepted as national documents from the Department of Education and were reinforced by assistance from the Education Officer, Nursing and Māori Health.

Origin of the term *cultural safety*

A first-year student from Te Arawa studying nursing at Christchurch Polytechnic was at the Hui Waimanawa. Although shy because of the status of other participants, she had been listening carefully to the talk and to the language being used. Finally she rose to her feet and said that legal safety, ethical safety, safe practice/clinical base and a safe knowledge base were all very well to expect from graduate nurses, *"but what about cultural safety?"*. This young woman was overwhelmed by her own courage. Sitting in the hui, I picked up what she said and with her permission from that time adopted the term *cultural safety* to refer to the work which has since emerged from the hui.

Acceptance by the Nursing Council of New Zealand and the schools offering nursing and midwifery education of the two documents, *A Model For Negotiated and Equal Partnership* (Ramsden, 1989a), and *Kawa Whakaruruhau: Cultural Safety in Nursing Education in Aotearoa* (Ramsden, 1990), legitimated the term *cultural safety* and admitted it to the nursing and midwifery lexicon. Linda Wilson, Head of School, Occupational Therapy, Otago

Polytechnic, and I (personal communication, Dunedin, 1993) identified expected educational outcomes of a culturally safe graduate health professional, as presented in Table 1.1.

TABLE 1.1 *Outcomes of a culturally safe health professional*

All graduates	develop the skills of critical analysis
All graduates	recognise where things are wrong
Two-thirds of graduates	recognise the opportunities to create change and see where to intervene
One-third of graduates	contribute to change
Outstanding graduates	initiate change

This is not a measure of any group of students at any time, but simply a model to which students and teachers may aspire. It does not require concrete prescription but rather creates a set of aims which students and teachers can see as achievable alongside their own rhythm and pace of development. It does not stipulate that students will have reached a prescribed level of achievement by a given time, but acknowledges the rate at which each student works and it also agrees that such learning may take place over a total lifetime, and that learning does not need to be confined to a three-year programme.

Moving into a teaching environment and having direct contact with students from the very beginning of their training gave me further insight into both my own and their learning needs about emancipatory change and ways in which this information could be approached and used meaningfully within nursing and midwifery.

To some extent, the key concepts of cultural safety education were already in place prior to my moving into teaching. However, there had been no education framework on which to 'hang' the concepts, learnt as a practitioner, which could be relevant to those students in a classroom who were without a practice base. The two components of theory and practice needed to be brought together for me as a teacher, and from that position I could bring the same information and analysis to students as they moved through their training and were exposed to practice situations.

The key objectives of *cultural safety* education arose directly from these practice/classroom encounters:

- to educate student nurses and midwives not to blame the victims of historical processes for their current plights;
- to educate student nurses and midwives to examine their own realities and the attitudes they bring to each new person they encounter in their practice;

- to educate student nurses and midwives to be open minded and flexible in their attitudes toward people who are different from themselves, to whom they offer and deliver service;
- to produce a workforce of well-educated, self-aware registered nurses and midwives who are culturally safe to practice, as defined by the people they serve.

These objectives formed the basis for the early *cultural safety* documents I produced to this day, the fundamental cornerstones on which cultural safety education is based.

References

Bell, L. (1992). *Colonial constructs: European images of Māori 1840–1914*. Auckland: Auckland University Press.

Bruni, N. (1988). A critical analysis of transcultural theory. *The Australian Journal of Advanced Nursing, 5*, 26–32.

Durie, M. (1989). The Treaty of Waitangi and health care. *New Zealand Medical Journal, 102*, 283–5.

Durie, M. (1994). *Whaiora: Māori health development*. Auckland: Oxford University Press.

Freire, P. (1996). *Pedagogy of the oppressed*. London: Penguin.

Johnstone, M.-J. & Ecker, M. (2001). Ethics and professional practice. In J. Crisp & C. Taylor (eds) *Potter and Perry's fundamentals of nursing*. Australian edn. Sydney: Mosby.

Lather, P. (1991). *Getting smart: Feminist research and pedagogy with/in the postmodern*. New York: Routledge.

Leininger, M. (1991). *Culture care diversity and universality: A theory of nursing*. New York: National League for Nursing Press.

National Action Group. (1988). *The aims and scope of nursing*. Wellington: National Action Group.

Nursing Council of New Zealand. (1994). *Strategic plan: 1994–1997*. Wellington: Nursing Council of New Zealand.

Nursing Council of New Zealand. (1996). *Guidelines for cultural safety in nursing and midwifery education*. Wellington: Nursing Council of New Zealand.

Papps, E. (2002). *Nursing in New Zealand: Critical issues, different perspectives*. Auckland: Pearson Education.

Pere, R. T. (1991). *Te Wheke. A celebration of infinite wisdom*. Gisborne: Ao Ako Global Publishing.

Ramsden, I. (1988). Graduation address. Paper given to graduating Diploma of Nursing class at Nelson Polytechnic, Nelson, November.

Ramsden, I. (1989a). *A model for negotiated and equal partnership.* Wellington: Author.

Ramsden, I. (1989b). Piri ki nga tangaroa: In anticipation of better days. Paper presented at the Health in Multicultural Societies Conference, Melbourne, September.

Ramsden, I. (1990). *Kawa Whakaruruhau: Cultural safety in nursing education in Aotearoa.* Wellington: Ministry of Education.

Ramsden, I. (2000). Cultural safety/Kawa whakaruruhau ten years on: A personal overview. *Nursing Praxis in New Zealand, 15*(1), 4–12.

Ramsden, I. & Spoonley, P. (1994). The cultural safety debate in nursing education in Aotearoa. *New Zealand Annual Review of Education 1993,* 161–74.

Royal Commission on Social Policy. (1988). *The April report.* Wellington: Royal Commission on Social Policy.

Shuker, R. (1987). *The One Best System? A revisionist history of state schooling in New Zealand.* Palmerston North: Dunmore.

Te Puni Kokiri. (2000). *Progress towards closing social and economic gaps between Māori and Non-Māori.* A report to the Minister of Māori Affairs. Wellington: Te Puni Kokiri.

Wetherell, M. & Potter, J. (1992). *Mapping the language of racism. Discourse and the legitimation of exploitation.* Brighton: Harvester Wheatsheaf.

Note

This chapter is an excerpt from Irihapeti Ramsden's PhD thesis (Chapters 5 and 6): *Cultural safety and nursing education in Aotearoa and Te Waipounamu* (2001). Reprinted with the permission of her whānau and Victoria University.

2 Cultural safety and the Nursing Council of New Zealand

Liz Banks and Maureen Kelly

Ki te whakarite i ngā ā huatanga o ngā Tapuhi e pā ana mo ngā iwi katoa

Regulating nursing practice to protect public safety

Learning objectives

Having studied this chapter, you will be able to:

- understand the role of the Nursing Council of New Zealand in relation to culturally safe nursing care;

- enhance your ability to reflect on nursing practice in relation to culturally safe nursing care;

- identify examples from practice to demonstrate how the Nursing Council of New Zealand competencies for the registered nurse's scope of practice for cultural safety and the Treaty of Waitangi may be met.

Key terms and concepts

- competencies

- cultural safety

- domains of competence

- Nursing Council of New Zealand

- scope of practice

- Treaty of Waitangi/Tiriti o Waitangi

Introduction

This chapter focuses primarily on the relationship between cultural safety, the Treaty of Waitangi, Māori health and the legislative requirements of the Nursing Council of New Zealand ('the Nursing Council'). This includes the ongoing requirements for enrolled nurses, registered nurses and nurse practitioners to demonstrate competence against the competencies for their designated scope of practice. Through the use of practice examples from a registered nurse and student nurse, we consider how nurses demonstrate competence in relation to cultural safety and the Treaty of Waitangi ('the Treaty'). The use of reflective questions at the end of each practice example enables you to consider your own practice and the examples that you may be able to draw from your practice to demonstrate competence.

Legislation and standards

Under the Health Practitioners Competence Assurance Act) 2003 ('the Act'), the Nursing Council governs the practice of nurses by setting and monitoring standards and competencies for registration which ensures safe and competent care for the public of New Zealand (Nursing Council of New Zealand, 2011a).

Cultural safety, the Treaty and Māori health are aspects of nursing practice that are reflected in the Nursing Council's Education Programme Standards for the Registered Nurse Scope of Practice ('the Standards'). The Standards for the registration of nurses require that the content of theory- and practice-related experience in nursing programmes include cultural safety, the Treaty and Māori health. Competencies outlined in the scopes of practice for nurses (Nursing Council of New Zealand, 2009, 2010) require the nurse to practise nursing in a manner that the client determines as being culturally safe and to demonstrate the ability to apply the principles of the Treaty to nursing practice. Additionally, the Nursing Council's Code of Conduct for Nurses (Nursing Council of New Zealand, 2012), requires nurses to respect the cultural needs and values of clients, and practise in compliance with the Treaty. Nurses are assessed against the competencies on an ongoing basis. As the regulatory authority, the Nursing Council is committed to enabling nursing workforce excellence.

Cultural safety

Cultural safety relates to the experience of the recipient of nursing care and extends beyond cultural awareness and cultural sensitivity (Nursing Council of New Zealand, 2011a). It provides clients with the power to comment on practices and contribute to the achievement of positive health outcomes and experiences. It also enables clients to participate in changing any negatively perceived or experienced service. The Nursing Council (Nursing Council of New Zealand, 2011b, p. 7) defines cultural safety as:

> The effective nursing practice of a person or family from another culture, and is determined by that person or family. Culture includes, but is not restricted to, age or generation; gender; sexual orientation; occupation and socioeconomic status; ethnic origin or migrant experience; religious or spiritual belief; and disability.

> The nurse delivering the nursing service will have undertaken a process of reflection on his or her own cultural identity and will recognise the impact that his or her personal culture has on his or her professional practice. Unsafe cultural practice comprises any action which diminishes, demeans or disempowers the cultural identity and well being of an individual.

Meeting the Nursing Council's competencies

Cultural safety is an integral component of the Nursing Council's competencies for registered nurses. Similar requirements are also expected of enrolled nurses and nurse practitioners. To demonstrate how the concepts are utilised, examples have been included from clinical and teaching practice. Competence is the combination of skills, knowledge, attitudes, values and abilities that underpin effective performance as a nurse. The Nursing Council has developed competencies that describe the skills and knowledge expected of nurses registered in each scope of practice. To practise safely, nurses are expected to demonstrate how they meet these competencies. Nurses are required to reflect on whether they meet these competencies yearly, at the time when they make their annual declaration as part of the process of applying for their annual practising certificate, and to be assessed against these competencies at least every three years.

Domains of competence

There are four domains of competence for the registered nurse's scope of practice: professional responsibility, management of nursing care, interpersonal relationships, and interprofessional health care and quality (Nursing Council of New Zealand, 2009). Evidence of safety to practise as a registered nurse is demonstrated when the competencies within the four domains are met. The competencies in each domain have a number of key generic examples of competence performance called indicators. These are neither comprehensive nor exhaustive; rather they provide examples of evidence of competence. The indicators are designed to assist assessors when using their professional judgement in assessing the attainment of the competencies. The indicators further assist curriculum development for bachelor degrees in nursing or first year of practice programmes.

Domain one 'professional responsibility' contains competencies that relate to professional, legal and ethical responsibilities, and cultural safety. These include being able to demonstrate knowledge and judgement, and being accountable for one's own actions and decisions, while promoting an environment that maximises client safety, independence, quality of life and health. Within this domain there are two competencies with 1.2 focusing on culturally safe practice with Māori and 1.5 applying the concepts of cultural safety to all relationships with health consumers.

In Competency 1.2, the Nursing Council recognises the status of Māori as the indigenous people of New Zealand and requires nurses to develop knowledge and understanding of the differing health outcomes of Māori and non-Māori, supporting equity by providing culturally safe nursing services with Māori. The Nursing Council requires nurses to demonstrate their ability to apply the principles of the Treaty to nursing practice and their ability to practise nursing in a manner that the client determines as being culturally safe. The Royal Commission on Social Policy (1988) identified the principles of partnership, protection, and participation which are 'drawn from both versions of the Treaty and are used to better understand how the Treaty may be applied' (Kingi, 2007, p. 8). It is an expectation that nurses will demonstrate these principles when providing nursing services with Māori.

- **Partnership:** working together with iwi, hapū, whānau and Māori communities to develop strategies for Māori health gain and appropriate health and disability services.
- **Participation:** involving Māori at all levels of the sector, in decision making, planning, development, and delivery of health and disability services.
- **Protection:** working to ensure Māori have at least the same level of health as non-Māori and safeguarding Māori cultural concepts, values and practices (Royal Commission on Social Policy, 1988).

Competency 1.2

Demonstrates the ability to apply the principles of the Treaty of Waitangi/Te Tiriti o Waitangi to nursing practice.

> **Indicator:** Understands the Treaty of Waitangi/Te Tiriti o Waitangi and its relevance to the health of Māori in Aotearoa New Zealand.

> **Indicator:** Demonstrates knowledge of differing health and socio-economic status of Māori and non-Māori.

> **Indicator:** Applies the Treaty of Waitangi/Te Tiriti o Waitangi to nursing practice.

(Nursing Council of New Zealand, 2009, p. 10)

In Competency 1.5, the Nursing Council requires nurses to practise in a culturally safe manner, as defined by the recipients of their care, with all clients. It is expected that these nurses will be competent in examining their own realities and the attitudes they bring to each new client that they encounter. They will be able to evaluate the impact that historical, political and social processes have on the health of all people and will be able to demonstrate flexibility in their relationships with people who are different from themselves (Nursing Council of New Zealand, 2011a).

Competency 1.5

Practises nursing in a manner that the client determines as being culturally safe.

> **Indicator:** Applies the principles of cultural safety in own nursing practice.

> **Indicator:** Recognises the impact of the culture of nursing on client care and endeavours to protect the client's well-being within this culture.

> **Indicator:** Practises in a way that respects each client's identity and right to hold personal beliefs, values and goals.

> **Indicator:** Assists the client to gain appropriate support and representation from those who understand the client's culture, needs and preferences.

> **Indicator:** Consults with members of cultural and other groups as requested and approved by the client.

> **Indicator:** Reflects on his/her own practice and values that impact on nursing care in relation to the client's age, ethnicity, culture, beliefs, gender, sexual orientation and/or disability.

> **Indicator:** Avoids imposing prejudice on others and provides advocacy when prejudice is apparent.

(Nursing Council of New Zealand, 2009, p. 13)

Other competencies describe generic skills which also relate to cultural safety, such as Competency 1.4, which states that nurses need to provide a suitable environment that best meets the needs and interests of the clients. In

Competency 2.4, nurses must ensure that clients have adequate explanations of the effect and possible consequence of treatment including alternative to proposed treatment options, with their preferences being included. This would require the nurses to be client-centred and to explore with the clients in a way they can understand.

Competency 2.6 identifies that nurses must evaluate clients' progress towards expected outcomes utilising partnership principles and Competency 3.1 refers to the importance of establishing, maintaining and concluding therapeutic inter-personal relationships. These relationships need to establish rapport and trust, and demonstrate respect, empathy and interest with the client. Competency 3.2 affirms that nurses must work in a negotiated partnership with clients where possible and acknowledge family and whānau perspectives. Nurses must communicate effectively, share information with clients and acknowledge their level of health literacy therefore enabling them to make informed choices. A range of communication techniques need to be employed by nurses, depending on the context, such as utilising interpreters and providing adequate time for discussions.

The following section provides two practice examples, one from the perspective of a registered nurse and the other from a student nurse. These practice examples provide a context for 'deconstructions of practice narratives' (McEldowney & Connor, 2011 p. 6) around how competencies can be met, and the subsequent reflection and discussion that needs to occur to demonstrate or determine competence in relation to cultural safety and the Treaty.

Hine and her baby

Practice example 1

This situation happened some years back when I worked as a telenurse and I have told this story as an educator on occasions to demonstrate a range of nursing concepts. Following the 'story', I will raise questions about my practice in relation to the demonstration of Competencies 1.2 and 1.5.

I received a call from a mother who was concerned about her baby's sleep. She explained to me that her eight-month-old baby girl would wake at about 11pm at night. She would get her up and play with her, and then, when the baby was tired, she would put her back to bed. I commented that this must make her tired and she said it did as she was pregnant again. I asked when the baby was due and worked out in my head that her next baby would arrive when this baby was 11 months old. She said that when her baby slept in the afternoon she did also, to help catch up on sleep. I commented on what an attentive mother she was to her daughter.

To make a fuller assessment around sleep, I asked about her baby's nutrition and if she was offering her meat as part of her diet. She said she didn't really know how to cook meat so, when I asked if she would like some information on how to cook meat for a baby, she indicated that she would. I shared information about the recommended ways and then she asked a question I was not expecting. She asked 'would it be all right to give her the inside of a mince pie?' I paused with a range of things going through my mind.

I sensed from her question that she may be a very young mother and that giving a baby mince from the inside of a pie would not be supported by evidence. I recognised, however, that there would be some iron content in the mince (even if there may be some less desirable ingredients for one so young), which the baby was not currently getting. I also recognised that this caller spoke so kindly of her baby, was so attentive to her baby's needs and seemed to be trying to do the best in the circumstances. I paused then responded, 'Yes, I suppose it would be OK' and we discussed again about how to cook other meats for her baby.

At the end of the phone call I asked her the demographic information required for statistical and funding purposes like her name, ethnicity and age. She said her name was Hine (changed to protect her identity), she was Māori and she was 16. The call was about to end but this new information added another dimension and I quickly asked her if she had support and she said 'Yes' and the call ended.

Following the call I felt troubled and empty. I questioned whether I had served Hine and her baby well – had I been sensitive and regardful of her particular needs? I felt concerned that I had not enquired into her support systems earlier and then, once I had, the discussion was only brief before the call ended.

This call weighed heavily on my mind and I realised that I had limited knowledge about younger parents, and the strengths and challenges that they face. I was undertaking a Master of Nursing at the time so devoted an assignment to understanding more about those who parent young.

(*Competency 1.2*)

> Did I apply the Treaty to my nursing practice and did I demonstrate the principles of partnership, protection and participation? Did I offer her or her baby protection by recognising that, as her baby was not having meat in her diet (a rich source of iron), she could become anaemic? (Ministry of Health, 2008). Did I demonstrate a partnership approach by asking her if she would like some information about cooking meat for her baby? Did I encourage or enable her to participate in the discussion we had around the health and well-being of her and her baby?

> Does this practice example demonstrate that I had an understanding of the Treaty and its relevance to the health of Hine and her baby? If so, what aspect? Did I ensure that the information shared was appropriate for Hine as a Māori mother whilst recognising that Māori are a diverse population?

> Did I acknowledge and work with her in a way that respected her ethnicity, age, education, and socio-economic status, whilst recognising that Māori have on average poorer health than non-Māori (Ministry of Health, 2002)?

(*Competency 1.5*)

> Did Hine, as the health consumer, find me and the information that I shared culturally safe? How would I as the provider of care know this? Could the fact that she was able to ask me the question about the mince pie imply that I had created a safe context for her to reveal what was important to her? Were we able to connect across our differences?

> Did I practise in a way that respected Hine's identity and her right to hold personal beliefs, values and goals? What could I have done to assess her goals and values? Did I recognise my own power and privilege and use it wisely? Was there anything in this story that demonstrated my competence?

> I did not assist Hine to gain appropriate support and representation from those who understand the client's culture, needs and preferences. When she said 'yes' to my closed question about support, I left it at that. If this situation arose again, how could I be more appropriate, relevant and supportive to Hine? What representation would a service require to ensure the service provided was sensitive to the needs of all who use it?

> I did undertake a process of reflection following the call and wondered how differently I may have worked with her if I had known that Hine was Māori and 16 years old at the start of the call. I did consider my own cultural identity and recognised that I did not want to impose my values on her (having been a by-the-book mother with my own children). I also recognised that there was an expectation that I would share evidence-based information as was expected with all callers.

> What strategies do we employ when we need to balance evidence-based practice with the needs and preferences of clients or their families or whānau?

> I believe that I did avoid imposing prejudices towards Hine and recognised that her circumstances were very different to my own. I was keen to recognise and comment to her about the sensitive, nurturing mother that she appeared to be and be strengths-based in my approach by recognising that she was a sensitive mother to her baby.

Jo and Martin

Practice example 2

Jo (name changed to protect her identity) was admitted to the orthopaedic ward for surgery to insert a 'portacath' to enable the easy administration of antibiotics to treat a persistent bone infection. This was the final stage of treatment for Jo, who had undergone a number of previous surgical procedures for injuries sustained in a car accident many months prior. Coming to hospital regularly for surgery was something Jo had come to dread and it appeared that some of the staff on the ward had also come to dread Jo's regular admissions. As a student nurse on a short placement on the orthopaedic ward, I chose not to explore the reasons why some staff felt negatively about Jo as I did not want to be influenced by

their reasons when it came to caring for her. For Jo and her partner Martin (name changed to protect his identity), there was a sense of expectation and hope that this surgery would be the final stage in Jo's recovery.

I asked to be involved in Jo's care and, if possible, to accompany her to theatre. As many of the staff on the ward were not keen to work with Jo, they were happy for me to take a major role in her care. Jo consented to my taking part in her care and also to my accompanying her to theatre. I worked with a registered nurse to prepare Jo for surgery. During the preparation, I chatted to Jo and Martin, asking them questions about previous surgeries and Jo's recovery from her accident. During this time I formed what I believed to be a therapeutic relationship with both Jo and Martin.

When the time came for Jo to go to theatre, I accompanied Jo and Martin down to the theatre entrance. When we got there Jo and Martin said their goodbyes and kissed. Martin then took Jo's hand out of his and placed it in my hand. He looked me in the eye and said to me 'You need to be there for me during Jo's surgery as I am not able to be'. Jo squeezed my hand tightly as Martin was saying this to me. It felt good that Martin had trusted me in this way. I felt that I had built a therapeutic relationship with this couple in a short space of time to the point where Martin felt comfortable to say and do what he did and for Jo to allow me to accompany her to theatre.

The surgery went according to plan and I was with Jo the whole time. I then stayed with her in recovery and accompanied her back to the ward. When we were back in the ward I spoke to Martin and in effect handed Jo back to him. The shift ended and I went home. When I returned for my next shift, Jo had been discharged from hospital.

While there have been many other stories from my nursing career that I could have relayed, this is one that has always stayed in my mind as it was a time when I believe I truly connected with someone I cared for. I felt I was able to develop, maintain and conclude a therapeutic relationship in a short space of time.

(*Competency 1.5*)

FOR REFLECTION

> How would you determine if Jo and Martin found that the care they were provided with was culturally safe? What might they say or do that would reassure you that they found the care culturally safe?

> How might the culture of nursing have impacted on Jo and Martin if they knew that other staff 'dreaded' Jo's visits? What effect may that have had on them? How, within nursing, do we protect clients from the possible negative effect of our culture such as labelling particular clients if they do not conform to how we want or expect them to behave? How can we break the cycle of labelling if it has become the culture in our workplace? What effect may the role modelling of this behaviour by registered nurses have on students? What might the barriers be for a student to speak up to protect the rights of the health consumer?

> How were Jo's and Martin's identities and rights to hold personal beliefs, values and goals upheld? What would we, as a nurse or a student nurse, do if personal beliefs, values and goals were not upheld by a colleague? Would we challenge them and, if not, what are the barriers?

> If Jo's and Martin's culture, needs and preferences differed to that of the 'student nurse', what supports or resources could a student access? How as a preceptor might we guide this process?

> How might a 'student' reflect on their own practice and values that may impact on nursing care in relation to the client's age, ethnicity, culture, beliefs, gender, sexual orientation and/or disability? How can we work with students to enable them to recognise their own culture and how it may influence the care they provide? As a student, if we conscientiously objected with the beliefs of a health consumer, how would we respond?

Conclusion

This chapter described how the Nursing Council, under the Act, regulates the practice of nurses. This occurs by setting and monitoring standards of competence for registration which ensures safe and competent nursing care for the public of New Zealand. Cultural safety has been defined by the Nursing Council with health consumers determining if the care provided is culturally safe. There are four domains of competence for the registered nurse scope of practice, with cultural safety being an integral component of these competencies.

We have provided two practice examples to aid discussion and reflection to enable students, registered nurses and nurse educators to critique how nursing practice may and may not demonstrate competence, and what constitutes evidence, particularly in the ability to apply the principles of the Treaty and cultural safety.

References

Kingi, T. R. (2007). The Treaty of Waitangi: A framework for Māori health development. *New Zealand Journal of Occupational Therapy, 54*(1), 4–10.

McEldowney, R. & Connor, M. J. (2011). Cultural safety as an ethic of care: A praxiological process. *Journal of Transcultural Nursing, 22*(4), 342–9. doi: 10.1177/1043659611414139

Ministry of Health. (2002). *He korowai oranga: Māori health strategy.* Wellington: Ministry of Health.

Ministry of Health. (2008). Food and nutrition guidelines for healthy infants and toddlers (Aged 0–2): A background paper (4th edn.). Wellington: Ministry of Health.

Nursing Council of New Zealand. (2009). *Competencies for registered nurses.* Wellington: Nursing Council of New Zealand.

Nursing Council of New Zealand. (2010). *Competencies for the enrolled nurse scope of practice.* Wellington: Nursing Council of New Zealand.

Nursing Council of New Zealand. (2011a). *Strategic plan 2011–2012.* Wellington: Nursing Council of New Zealand.

Nursing Council of New Zealand. (2011b). *Guidelines for cultural safety, the Treaty of Waitangi and Māori health in nursing education and practice.* Wellington: Nursing Council of New Zealand.

Nursing Council of New Zealand. (2012). *Code of conduct for nurses.* Wellington: Nursing Council of New Zealand.

Royal Commission on Social Policy. (1988). *The April report.* Royal Commission on Social Policy, 3(1), 24–32.

3 Cultural safety DARING TO BE DIFFERENT

Elaine Papps

Learning objectives

Having studied this chapter, you will be able to:

- describe the history of nursing in relation to cultural safety;

- understand the difference between cultural sameness (transcultural nursing) and cultural difference (cultural safety);

- describe the structural patterns and power dynamics within nursing.

Key terms and concepts

- cultural awareness

- cultural safety

- cultural sensitivity

- dominant discourse

- power relationships

- respect for difference

- transcultural nursing

Introduction

There was a time in my life when I almost wished I had never heard of cultural safety, let alone have any part in its introduction into nursing and midwifery education curricula. Between October 1990 and May 1996, I chaired the Nursing Council of New Zealand ('the Nursing Council'). During that time, cultural safety was a major and extraordinarily contentious issue. The Nursing Council's resolution that cultural safety would be part of the requirements for nursing and midwifery education programmes might be considered as one of the greatest challenges to face the nursing profession in New Zealand.

My experiences at the time cultural safety was introduced were intensely personal and highly political, and at times, my professional values were compromised.

However, my interest in issues of power and knowledge, particularly in relation to nursing in New Zealand society, enabled me to reflect on and analyse some of the reasons why cultural safety was subjected to aggressive questioning by journalists, politicians and members of the public. This chapter provides a personal analysis of why cultural safety was almost lost from the language of nursing. It begins with a brief historical perspective on nursing and cultural safety in New Zealand. The important differences between transcultural nursing and cultural safety are discussed, as well as the ensuing public debate that followed cultural safety's early development.

Nursing's background

It is useful, as a way of setting the scene, to look at the place of nurses and nursing education in New Zealand from a brief historical perspective. Nursing's history is steeped in tradition and throughout history nurses have been shaped and positioned in a particular way, essentially because of beliefs about what they do and what they need to know.

Although there is no definitive book to turn to in order to read about the history of nursing and nursing education in New Zealand, a number of publications, such as articles in nursing journals, chapters in books, and academic theses, offer this information. Most writers acknowledge that nursing developed in New Zealand in the late 1870s and 1880s, when nurses who had trained at Florence Nightingale's School for Nurses in London came to New Zealand to help improve the standard of hospital services (Papps, 1997).

In 1901, the enactment of legislation in New Zealand to register nurses introduced:

- a standard curriculum;
- a national examination that all student nurses needed to pass in order to be registered nurses;
- the concept of nurses becoming a legal entity.

For around 70 years, the training of nurses was undertaken in hospital schools of nursing, where the substantial part of training happened 'on the job', although nursing students attended lectures during study days or block courses. But nursing students also provided patient care within a strict hierarchical structure. They were distinctive in their various uniforms over this period of time; their position in the hierarchy identified by symbols, such as stripes on uniform sleeves or caps, as they proceeded through their three-year training period, mostly in hospitals and as 'general' nurses.

When the system of nursing education began to change during the 1970s, moving from hospital schools of nursing into the tertiary education system, the status of student nurses changed from being employees of an organisation paid to learn nursing while providing service, to students within the education system. The new system of nursing education shifted to student-based learning and prepared individuals for a new category of registration – comprehensive registration. Nurses were now being prepared to provide care in a variety of health settings.

This change, it can be argued, challenged a perception of nursing and nurses interlinked with Florence Nightingale's legacy of duty, obedience and servitude. A further disruption to this perception came about with the introduction of undergraduate nursing degrees in the early 1990s. The literature at this time reflects uncertainty that 'educated' nurses would ever be able to acquire the skills necessary to undertake the complexities of hands-on patient care. The dominant view of nurses as doers rather than thinkers suggested that not all registered nurses needed to be educated to degree level.

The introduction of cultural safety to nursing and midwifery education curricula coincided with the enactment of the Nurses Amendment Act 1990 and the commencement of three undergraduate degrees in nursing. It is noteworthy that although cultural safety was part of nursing and midwifery curricula, the ensuing scrutiny focused on nursing rather than on midwifery. A possible explanation for this could be a belief that nursing and midwifery were the same profession, even though this had been strongly contested for several years (Papps & Olssen, 1997).

Sameness and silencing

'Cultural safety' is a New Zealand term unique to nursing. It was born from the pain of the Māori experience of poor health care and evolved over 12 years against a backdrop of bicultural development. The Treaty of Waitangi ('the Treaty') provides the framework for its progression, which emphasises shifting power in the healthcare arena from nurses to those receiving care. Once this transfer of power has occurred, the recipients of care are empowered to define what is culturally safe practice. In other words, the 'lived experience' of patients determines whether or not a nurse is safe to attend to their cultural needs (Wepa, 2001).

By contrast, transcultural nursing, cultural safety's American predecessor, emerged from a multicultural context. Here, the emphasis is on 'cultural sensitivity' when dealing with patients with no consideration of a power imbalance in the healthcare setting. The focus is on the 'cultural' activities of the patient with no analysis of power (Ramsden, 2001). Its anthropological framework advocates the study of 'exotic' cultures where the health professional is considered acultural and normal. From these different beginnings the subsequent journeys that cultural safety and transcultural nursing have travelled remain disassociated.

The journey of transcultural nursing began in the United States in the 1950s, when Madeline Leininger, a nurse theorist then working in a child guidance home, recognised the need to respond to people from diverse cultures. The context at the time was turbulent, as many wars and famine provided the catalyst for mass migration to the United States. This created an increase in legal suits for cultural negligence in the healthcare system (Leininger, 1995). The predominantly white American nursing profession possessed limited knowledge of different cultures. A small core of nurse leaders recognised this deficit and developed transcultural courses to deal with the influx of immigrants (Leininger, 1997). Leininger began the first transcultural nursing course in 1966 and gained credibility through her research into over 45 cultures using predominantly qualitative methods. She believed that transcultural nursing was essentially based on nurses having a scientific knowledge base about a range of different cultures from which they can respond therapeutically to their clients' needs (Leininger, 1997).

In 1970 she published her first book, *Nursing and Anthropology: Two Worlds to Blend*, which was instrumental in incorporating anthropology into many nursing programmes. Hence race relations began to be discussed, in elementary terms, in nursing. This was demonstrated by the transformation from nineteenth-century ethnocentrism towards the acknowledgement of the existence of cultural difference. Over the next 20 years, Leininger published many more books and papers which made her an authority on transcultural nursing care. In 1984 Leininger theorised that there could not be curing without caring. This theme remained throughout her literature: being human was to be caring and caring was culturally based (Reynolds & Leininger, 1993). This philosophy became interpreted as 'universal care' given irrespective of colour, code or creed, which was transposed into New Zealand nursing and midwifery education (Pere, 1997). Hospital Boards emphasised the theory that people should receive care without regard to their sex, race, or culture or their economic, educational or religious backgrounds (Nursing Council of New Zealand, 1996, p. 10). In 1995, at the time cultural safety was being debated in the media, a registered nurse endorsed this commonly held view in a letter to the Editor of the Christchurch *Press*:

> At Westminster Hospital in London I cared for patients from wide cultural backgrounds, including English aristocracy and Arabs from the United Arab Emirates. Not once did I transgress in the care of my patients due to my lack of so-called cultural sensitivity. (Cooke, 1995, p. 2)

The biblical premise of 'doing unto others as you would have done to you', which aimed to give care to all people as of right, in reality negated individual and cultural differences. The emphasis was firmly placed on the view of the nurse, rather than on that of the recipient of care. The dominance of transcultural nursing developed by Leininger (1991) became part of the struggle to retain cultural safety as something different and unique to New Zealand. Despite the efforts of various writers to differentiate between cultural safety and transcultural nursing (Cooney, 1994; Coup, 1996), there remained an apparent political agenda to have cultural safety renamed as something it clearly was not. Alternative concepts offered included cultural sensitivity, cultural awareness and cultural competence which are positioned within the dominant discourse of transcultural nursing.

The following figure describes the differences in meaning between these commonly used terms.

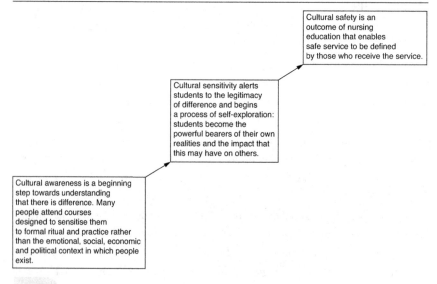

Cultural safety is an outcome of nursing education that enables safe service to be defined by those who receive the service.

Cultural sensitivity alerts students to the legitimacy of difference and begins a process of self-exploration: students become the powerful bearers of their own realities and the impact that this may have on others.

Cultural awareness is a beginning step towards understanding that there is difference. Many people attend courses designed to sensitise them to formal ritual and practice rather than the emotional, social, economic and political context in which people exist.

FIGURE 3.1   *The process towards achieving cultural safety in nursing practice*
Source: Adapted from the Nursing Council of New Zealand (2011, p. 4)

This curriculum staircase or poutama assumes that students begin their cultural safety education at the bottom of the staircase where they bring with them personal experience, knowledge and biases (Wood &d Schwass, 1993). Over the next three years of their education, the students are assessed on their ability to move to each next step with a focus on racism awareness, the Treaty, nga mea Māori (matters pertaining to Māori), and strategies for institutional change. Hence the educational process involves movement from sensitivity to awareness and, ultimately, to safety.

Prior to the introduction of the guidelines, Māori health professionals began challenging the lack of 'cultural dimension' in health programmes. Thus, the journey towards the inclusion of cultural safety in nursing education had begun. Durie (1994) provides a comprehensive overview of key events which include recommendations from The Board of Health Standing Committee on Māori Health made at a national conference in 1985. The recommendations addressed three levels of health training in New Zealand:

- Level 1, recommended for all New Zealand health professionals, was to provide educational opportunities to develop an understanding of the significance of culture on health practices and health services.
- Level 2 was seen as an introduction to Māori language and culture for all health students but without any expectation of high levels of proficiency.
- Level 3 was directed at students likely to work in Māori communities and who would therefore require a greater knowledge of Māori society, language and culture (Durie, 1994, p. 116).

The recommendations provided one of the first statements on a national level that recognised culture as an important influence on people's health. Unfortunately, the recommendations did not provide specific strategies on how health professionals would develop an understanding of the significance of culture on health. Nurse educators lacked training in this new dimension in health care and failed to provide a clear definition of culture to students. Culture, therefore, was equated with ethnicity which, in turn, translated into 'things Māori' (Papps & Ramsden, 1996). Nursing students were subsequently taught Māori words and songs instead of learning about their own cultural identity (Du Chateau, 1992).

Therefore, the second level of the recommendations – which stressed the introduction of Māori language and culture – became confusing as culture had not been clearly defined and there was no justification for its inclusion in relation to nursing practice. Subsequently, a National Action Group, which was formed in 1986, set the scene for further development of cultural safety education. Over the next three years, it held several hui and focused on extending the Board of Health's views on cultural training, and also advocated for the inclusion of politics and the Treaty (Durie, 1994).

Controversy and confusion

Compared with generalised nursing knowledge (such as medical and surgical knowledge), cultural safety knowledge, in its early days, was in an adolescent phase of development. This process has parallels with New Zealand's struggle to be considered a nation in its own right and not simply one of Britain's antipodean ex-colonies. Therefore, the controversy and confusion surrounding the development and definition of cultural safety was not unexpected. Several hui held in the late 1980s and early 1990s debated a variety of definitions. These included the following statements:

- Any actions which diminish, demean or disempower the cultural identity and well-being of an individual are defined as culturally unsafe.
- Culturally safe practice, therefore, would meet the following criteria: actions which recognise, respect and nurture the unique cultural identity of tangata whenua, and safely meet their needs, expectations and rights (Whānau Kawa Whakaruruhau, 1991).

The term became more clearly articulated to encompass a shift in power to the client, and cultural safety was originally defined by the Nursing Council in 1992 as:

> The effective nursing of a person/family from another culture by a nurse who has undertaken a process of reflection on own cultural identity and recognises the impact of the nurse's culture on own nursing practice. Unsafe cultural practice is any action which diminishes, demeans or disempowers the cultural identity and well-being of an individual. (Nursing Council of New Zealand, 1992, p. 1, glossary)

Cultural safety is based on attitudes which are difficult to measure. It needs to be considered alongside other equally important safety requirements such as clinical, ethical, legal and physical safety. Ethical safety, for example, requires students to provide appropriate responses in relation to individual events and to be based on the less measurable dimension of attitude. Cultural safety considerations are similar in that students are interacting in a bicultural (two-personed) context, where they are the giver of a health service and the client is the receiver of that service. These bicultural interactions will be different with every interaction but the nurse's awareness of the power differential between themselves and client will be constant.

This focus on power dynamics in health care and nursing education introduced a new form of knowledge for student nurses. Rightly or wrongly, the public believed that if new knowledge was to be introduced, then what would be omitted from the curriculum? Questions focused on the content and number of hours of 'nursing' in relation to the number of hours of cultural safety. There were claims that cultural safety had replaced more traditional knowledge content, such as 'medical' knowledge, and it was extravagantly claimed that this produced deficiencies in graduates of comprehensive nursing courses and made it difficult for them to be accepted in overseas countries (Papps & Ramsden, 1996).

This fuelled a developing public belief that the preparation of nurses for registration was inadequate, and that the Nursing Council was failing in its public duty to ensure adequate standards of education for nurses. Had these been factually accurate, there would have been cause for concern that nursing education was not adequately preparing student nurses for eventual registration as nurses.

Media attention over this issue fermented over a three-year period. Several commentators noted a number of themes that emerged from cultural safety's trial by media. First, Ramsden and Spoonley (1993) argued that members of the dominant cultural group in New Zealand were portrayed as victims of political correctness and appeared to have been disadvantaged in some way.

Second, the use of racist language in the media discredited Māori protest through labels such as 'activist' and 'militant'. Similarly, cultural safety was depicted as politically inspired while the curriculum of clinical nursing practice was apolitical and neutral. One of the ironies, therefore, has been the suggestion that, in an attempt to have cultural considerations examined, it became portrayed as an attempt to undermine critical and open debate. Jackson expands on this analysis and states that:

> Indeed, one of the ironies of the cultural safety debate has been that its advocates have been labelled as politically correct (one of the most ridiculing of today's labels) when for more than 150 years the correct political stance was to assert that race relations here were great and colonisation was somehow benign and humane. (Jackson, 1996, p. 10)

Third, the reasons why cultural safety is considered important by health professionals has seldom been given much attention. Similarly, the poor health status of Māori and the disease to which Māori were subjected when accessing services was underplayed in favour of the view that Māori were seeking more than were the rest of the population. According to Ramsden (1995, p. 6) 'the underlying issue was the apparent power of Māori to create meaningful change in an established Pākehā institution'.

Within these themes, images and vocabulary that were media-driven raised questions about Pākehā and Māori identity. New Zealand had always maintained the myth that its race relations were fundamentally good. But this was now being challenged as 'the heart of the colonial beast had been disturbed by a little part of an educational curriculum' (Jackson, 1996, p. 10).

On 25 July 1995, a member of the New Zealand Parliament, who chaired the Education and Science Select Committee of Parliament, announced in a press release that there was to be an enquiry into the cultural safety component of nursing education curricula. This press release stated there was:

> ...justification to hold such an enquiry to address this complex and contentious issue from the enormous number of public expressions of concern I have received and the correspondence generated on this matter. Clearly, there is more than enough support in the community for such an investigation to take place with many people believing that it is long overdue. (Bickley, 1998, p. 25)

Explanations around the time of the select committee hearings about cultural safety often focused on what it wasn't, rather than what it was (Papps, 2002). Justification for its inclusion in nursing education pointed out that, traditionally, nurses were educated not to recognise people's differences in the provision of nursing care, but to treat them all the same, while cultural safety was a way of caring for people recognising and respecting difference (Ramsden, 1995).

Several recommendations were made as a result of the enquiry. They included:

- the need to develop consistent curricula;
- the need for teachers to be skilled in facilitation and conflict resolution;
- the need to address the confusion between Māori studies and cultural safety in nursing education (Nursing Council of New Zealand, 1996, p. 6).

The Nursing Council also made a stand on two principles. They were:

1 the name 'cultural safety' would not be changed;
2 the Treaty of Waitangi would remain the basis for nursing education.

The culmination of these recommendations and principles resulted in the *Guidelines for Cultural Safety Component in Nursing and Midwifery* (1996), and subsequent guidelines, reviewed and published several times afterwards, the latest version published in 2011 (Nursing Council of New Zealand, 2011). Over this time cultural safety, the Treaty of Waitangi and Māori health have been clearly separated and the definition of cultural safety has been modified so that now it is defined as:

> the effective nursing practice of a person or family from another culture, and is determined by that person or family. Culture includes, but is not restricted to, age or generation; gender; sexual orientation; occupation and socioeconomic status; ethnic origin or migrant experience; religious or spiritual belief; and disability. The nurse delivering the service will have undertaken a process of reflection on his or her own cultural identity and will recognise the impact that his or her personal culture has on his or her professional practice. Unsafe cultural practice comprises any action which diminishes, demeans or disempowers the cultural identity and well being of an individual. (Nursing Council of New Zealand, 2011, p. x)

Knowledge, difference and power

While it must be acknowledged that there was controversy and confusion about the meaning of cultural safety when it was initially introduced into nursing education, it can be argued that one reason for this is that cultural safety did not sit within 'traditional' views about nurses and nursing knowledge. As identified earlier, nursing has had a long history of being trained in an apprenticeship system with the emphasis on the acquisition of technical skills or the 'doing' component of nursing. Although changes have occurred in the way that nurses are prepared for registration, there remains 'a residual ethos that the process of becoming a nurse is more about exposure to large quantities of clinical experience than about undertaking intellectual activity' (Papps & Kilpatrick, 2002, p. 11).

However, technical knowledge is only one part of the knowledge base for nurses. Habermas (1987), for example, asserts that there are 'knowledge-constitutive interests' – technical, interpretive, and emancipatory interests – which are distinct but interrelated domains of knowledge and each has a legitimate place in the world. Of note is that the emancipatory domain aims to bring about self-knowledge and self-reflection which are increasingly important in nursing education and practice. Attempts to subjugate some types of knowledge or exclude 'different' knowledge from nursing education privileges other knowledge, and raises an important question in terms of who decides what is appropriate for the language of nursing.

Researchers in Canada have commented that cultural safety will continue to hold value for nursing practice, research and education when used to emphasise critical self-reflection, critique of structures, discourses, power relations and assumptions, and because of its attachment to a social justice agenda (Browne et al., 2009, p. 177).

Conclusion

Cultural safety's focus on nursing people needs to be extended to respecting differences among and between health professional colleagues. To have it included in the education of others may assist the recognition that cultural safety is primarily about difference, respect for difference, power relationships between people, and the fundamental basic human rights of respect, dignity, safety, autonomy and empowerment.

The public and political debate about the relevance of cultural safety for nursing education, and the attempts to marginalise it, was a salutary lesson in how power is exercised in the development of new knowledge. The irony in the struggle to retain cultural safety in nursing education, as a means to empower clients to feel safe about that difference being recognised and respected, is that it was not respected for its difference. Intolerance towards difference was exemplified. My experiences, between 1993 and 1996 in particular, taught me a great deal about attitudes toward difference. It would have been easier at times to succumb to pressure to amalgamate the whole idea of cultural safety with that of transcultural nursing. But nurses dared to be different, raised their professional voice, and were strong and confident in the face of adversity.

References

Bickley, J. (1998). What's ahead for nursing? *Kai Tiaki Nursing New Zealand*, December/January, 24–5.

Browne, A. J., Varcoe, C., Smye, V., Reimer-Kirkham, S., Lyman, M. J. & Wong, S. (2009). Cultural safety and the challenges of translating critically oriented knowledge in practice. *Nursing Philosophy, 10*, 167–9.

Cooke, A. (1995). 'Cultural emphasis'. *The Press*, 3 July, 2.

Cooney, C. (1994). A comparative analysis of transcultural nursing and cultural safety. *Nursing Praxis in New Zealand, 9*, 6–12.

Coup, A. (1996). Cultural safety and culturally congruent care: A comparative analysis of Irihapeti Ramsden's and Madeleine Leininger's educational projects for practice. *Nursing Praxis in New Zealand, 11*(1), 4–11.

Du Chateau, C. (1992). Culture shock. *Metro*, June, 96–106.

Durie, M. (1994). *Whaiora: Māori health development*. Auckland: Oxford University Press.

Habermas, J. (1987). *Knowledge and human interests*, translated by J. Shapiro. Cambridge: Polity Press.

Jackson, M. (1996). Helping shape the wellbeing of a people. *Kia Hiwa Ra*, September, 10.

Leininger, M. (1991). *Cultural care diversity and universality: A theory for nursing*. New York: National League for Nursing.

Leininger, M. (1995). *Transcultural nursing concepts, theories, research and practices* (2nd edn.). New York: McGraw-Hill.

Leininger, M. (1997). Transcultural nursing research to transform nursing education and practice: 40 years. *Journal of Nursing Scholarship, 29*(4), 341–7.

Nursing Council of New Zealand. (1992). *Guidelines for the cultural safety component in nursing and midwifery education*. Wellington: Nursing Council of New Zealand.

Nursing Council of New Zealand. (1996). *Guidelines for the cultural safety component in nursing and midwifery education*. Wellington: Nursing Council of New Zealand.

Nursing Council of New Zealand. (2011). *Guidelines for cultural safety, the Treaty of Waitangi and Māori health in nursing education and practice*. Wellington: Nursing Council of New Zealand.

Papps, E. (1997). *Knowledge and power in nursing education in New Zealand: A critical analysis of the construction of the nursing identity*. Doctor of Philosophy thesis, University of Otago, Dunedin.

Papps, E. (2002). Cultural safety: What is the question? In E. Papps (ed.) *Nursing in New Zealand: Critical issues, different perspectives*. Auckland: Pearson Education New Zealand.

Papps, E. & Kilpatrick, J. (2002). Nursing education in New Zealand – past, present and future. In E. Papps (ed.) *Nursing in New Zealand: Critical issues, different perspectives*. Auckland: Pearson Education New Zealand.

Papps, E. & Olssen, M. (1997). *The doctoring of childbirth and the regulation of midwifery: A Foucauldian perspective*. Palmerston North: Dunmore.

Papps, E. & Ramsden, I. (1996). Cultural safety in nursing education: the New Zealand experience. *International Journal for Quality in Health Care, 8*(5), 491–7.

Pere, L. (1997). A study of kawa whakaruruhau/cultural safety education and its effects on the nursing practice of recently graduated registered comprehensive nurses. A thesis submitted in partial fulfilment of the requirements for the degree of Master of Arts (Applied) in Social Sciences Research, Victoria University, Wellington.

Ramsden, I. (1995). Cultural safety: Implementing the concepts. Paper presented at the Social Force of Nursing Conference, 23 May.

Ramsden, I. (2001). Improving practice through research. *Kai Tiaki Nursing New Zealand,* February, 23–6.

Ramsden, I. & Spoonley, P. (1993). The cultural safety debate in nursing education in Aotearoa. *New Zealand Annual Review of Education, 3,* 161–73.

Reynolds, C. & Leininger, M. (1993). *Madeleine Leininger: Cultural care diversity theory.* Newbury Park, CA: Sage.

Wepa, D. (2001). An exploration of the experiences of cultural safety educators. A thesis presented in partial fulfilment of the requirements for the degree of Master of Philosophy in Social Work, Massey University, Palmerston North.

Whānau Kawa Whakaruruhau. (1991). *Cultural safety hui of the Whānau Kawa Whakaruruhau.* Rotorua: Apumoana Marae.

Wood, P. & Schwass, M. (1993). Cultural safety: A framework for changing attitudes. *Nursing Praxis in New Zealand, 18*(1), 4–15.

part 2

The foundations of cultural safety

Cultural safety and continuing competence

4

Rachael Vernon and Elaine Papps

Learning objectives

Having studied this chapter, you will be able to:

- identify the requirements of the Health Practitioners Competence Assurance Act 2003 for health practitioners in New Zealand to demonstrate competence to practise;

- critically reflect on the difference between cultural competence and cultural safety;

- identify issues in the assessment of competence and continuing competence;

- explore how regulatory authorities in New Zealand address cultural competence in competence requirements;

- discuss how cultural safety and cultural competence is assessed in relation to demonstrating continuing competence.

Key terms and concepts

- competence

- continuing competence

- continuing competence framework

- cultural safety

- Health Practitioners Competence Assurance Act 2003

Introduction

In this chapter we explore the notions of competence, cultural safety and cultural competence, and analyse the way in which nurses in New Zealand are currently assessed to determine if they meet these requirements. As cultural safety had its origins in nursing education, this chapter has a primary focus on nursing. The introduction of cultural safety into nursing education curricula in New Zealand is well documented (Papps & Ramsden, 1996; Wepa, 2001; Papps,

2002a, Papps, 2005). The subsequent history of the journey of cultural safety has also recently been published (Nursing Council of New Zealand, 2013). Demonstration of competence is, however, a later requirement for all registered health practitioners, including nurses. We discuss this in relation to the requirements of the Health Practitioners Competence Assurance Act 2003 ('the Act').

In 1992 the Nursing Council of New Zealand ('the Nursing Council'), the regulatory authority for nursing in New Zealand, developed and published guidelines for nursing education curricula. Providers of nursing education courses were subsequently required to utilise these guidelines to include cultural safety into nursing courses leading to registration. Individuals completing a nursing education programme for registration as a nurse were subsequently required to demonstrate that they met cultural safety criteria on order to become registered nurses (Papps, 2002b). There was no requirement for registered nurses already practising to meet these criteria until the enactment of the Act. The Act requires regulatory authorities to 'set standards of clinical competence, cultural competence, and ethical conduct to be observed by health practitioners of the profession' (s 118(i)). This means that all registered health practitioners must now demonstrate that they are clinically competent and safe to practice, as well as meet a standard of cultural competence.

The key aspects of this chapter include a brief introduction to the Act and its relationship to competence, and an overview of continuing competence frameworks and the specific requirements of the Nursing Council in relation to competence. Issues around the notions of competence and continuing competence are explored, and finally there is a discussion about the cultural competence requirements of the Act.

The Health Practitioners Competence Assurance Act 2003

Nursing has been regulated in New Zealand for more than 100 years. However, the Act 2003 introduced significant change to the regulation of all health practitioners in New Zealand, including nurses (Vernon, 2014). Before the Act was introduced, there were 13 regulatory authorities and 11 separate statutes regulating 15 health professional groups in New Zealand (Vernon, 2013). None of these statutes required health practitioners to demonstrate that they were competent to practise or indeed to continue to practise. An annual practising certificate was issued simply on the basis of submitting an application form and paying the required fee (Papps, 2002b; Vernon et al., 2011). The Act changed that, as it has a clear focus on competence. The purpose of this Act is:

> to protect the health and safety of members of the public by providing for mechanisms to ensure that health practitioners are competent and fit to practice their professions. (Health Practitioners Competence Assurance Act 2003, s 10)

There are now 16 regulatory authorities, and each is authorised to develop its own systems and processes to meet the requirements of the Act. Additionally, each regulatory authority must specify and gazette the scope of practice for health practitioners under its jurisdiction and identify the qualifications for each scope (Health Practitioners Competence Assurance Act 2003, s 12). The Nursing Council has specified and gazetted three scopes of practice, each with their own registration and competence requirements. These are: registered nurse, enrolled nurse and nurse practitioner. Within each scope of practice, domains of practice and underpinning competencies are specified. All nurses registered under these scopes of practice must meet the specified standard of competence and continuing competence in order to be registered and to be issued an annual practising certificate.

The Act gives regulatory authorities significant power in relation to professional competence and requires that they 'set standards of clinical competence, cultural competence, and ethical conduct to be observed by health practitioners of the profession' (Health Practitioners Competence Assurance Act 2003, s 118(i)). These aspects are considered essential for health professional education and are concerned with the overarching notion of public protection, which are of equal significance under the Act 3 (s 4(6)). Competence is not defined in the Act but is considered to be a legislative function and, as such, is delegated to each of the regulatory authorities. Interpretation and enactment of the legislation in terms of demonstrating competence and continuing competence varies considerably between the different regulatory authorities in New Zealand.

The following section provides an overview of how the Nursing Council has addressed competence and continuing competence requirements, through the development of a continuing competence framework for nurses.

Continuing competence frameworks

A continuing competence framework (CCF) is a quality assurance mechanism designed to monitor and ensure that health professionals are and continue to be competent to practise, thereby providing a level of assurance to clients and employers (Australian Nursing and Midwifery Council, 2007; Canadian Nurses Association, 2000; Goodridge, 2007). These activities also provide a mechanism for identifying those who are not competent. Additionally, CCFs have an important function in regulating and guiding the profession (Australian Nursing and Midwifery Council, 2007; Bryant, 2005; Canadian Nurses Association, 2000) and ensure that there is consistency in the monitoring and ongoing assessment of competence standards.

The Nursing Council is the regulatory authority responsible for setting the education and registration standards for nurses in New Zealand. In 2004 the Nursing Council established and implemented a national CCF (Nursing Council of New Zealand, 2004) for nurses. The requirement that the Nursing Council implement a mechanism to ensure that nurses are competent and fit to practise their profession is a requirement stipulated in the Act. This new requirement meant there was a significant change to the process for nurses to renew their annual practising certificate. As noted earlier, the only requirement under the previous legislation that regulated nurses in New Zealand (Nurses Act 1977) was for nurses to renew their annual practising certificate by paying the annual fee and completing an application form. As noted earlier in this chapter, there was no requirement for a nurse to declare competence, to provide evidence of being competent (Papps, 1997) or indeed for the Nursing Council to monitor a practitioner's continuing competence.

With the responsibility for the ongoing monitoring of the continuing competence of nurses, the Nursing Council can now decline to issue an annual practising certificate if the applicant has, at any time, failed to meet the required standard of competence, failed to comply with conditions, not completed an ordered competence programme or not held an annual practising certificate (or been practising as a nurse) for three years preceding application (Health Practitioners Competence Assurance Act 2003, s 12(4)). The 'required standard of competence' is defined as 'the standard of competence reasonably to be expected of a health practitioner practising within that health practitioner's scope of practice' (Health Practitioners Competence Assurance Act 2003, s 5(1)). The Nursing Council has defined competence as 'the combination of skills, knowledge, attitudes, values and abilities that underpin effective performance as a nurse' (Nursing Council of New Zealand, 2010a).

Since there is no definition of competence or indeed continuing competence provided in the Act, and in order to determine whether a nurse requires an annual practising certificate in terms of employment, the Nursing Council has defined what practising nursing is. This definition states that a nurse:

> is using nursing knowledge in a direct relationship with clients or working in nursing management, nursing administration, nursing research, nursing professional advice or nursing policy development roles, which impact on public safety. (Nursing Council of New Zealand, 2010b)

When a nurse receives an annual practising certificate renewal form, a declaration must be signed that the competencies for whichever scope of practice the nurse is registered in have been met. The current CCF requirements are that nurses must provide evidence in three areas. First there has to be evidence of ongoing professional practice, which is stated as:

> nursing practice in a capacity for which a nursing qualification is required in order to practise in direct relationship with clients, or in nursing management and administration, nursing education, nursing research or nursing professional advice or policy development – minimum of 60 days or 450 hours within the last three years. (Nursing Council of New Zealand, 2006, p. 4)

Second, there has to be evidence of ongoing professional development. The requirement for this is a minimum of 60 hours in the last three years, relevant to work environment and practice as a nurse. The third requirement is providing evidence of meeting the Nursing Council's competencies for the nurse's scope of practice. This involves a self-declaration that states individuals meet the competencies for their particular scope of practice (Nursing Council of New Zealand, 2006).

Five per cent of nurses are selected for recertification audit annually. This is a random audit and, when nurses receive their annual practising certificate renewal information, they are advised at that time if they will be audited. Nurses can be exempt from audit if they participate in a professional development and recognition programme (PDRP) which has been approved by the Nursing Council (Nursing Council of New Zealand, 2004). These programmes are administered by health employer groups, such as District Health Boards. Those nurses who choose to participate in a PDRP approved by Nursing Council have a portfolio which is assessed within their employing organisation. Nurses who choose not to participate or do not have access to a PDRP are subject to selection by the Nursing Council in the random recertification audit process.

While there is a legal mandate in New Zealand for regulatory authorities to have processes in place to meet the requirements of the Act, many countries internationally have similar mechanisms, however continuing competence requirements are not consistent internationally. What is important to understand, though, is that various organisations have different roles and responsibilities in relation to the nursing profession, that is, individual nurses, employers, regulatory authorities and professional organisations. It is evident from current literature that, although individual nurses are responsible and accountable for their own competence and maintaining continuing competence, employers have also responsibility in terms of identifying, facilitating and supporting continued competence in the workplace (Vernon et al., 2010; Vernon, 2013). Employers have a role in ensuring that nurses hold a current practising certificate, are employed in a position that is appropriate to their scope of practice, and are supported and performance managed in their workplace. Regulatory authorities have responsibility for the quality assurance mechanisms that monitor and ensure nurses meet specific competence requirements. The next section outlines some of the issues associated with assessing continuing competence.

Assessment of continuing competence

Assessing the competence of practising nurses is an important part of maintaining professional standards and as such has a role in professional regulation (Chiarella et al., 2008). However, there is no international consensus about the meaning of continuing competence, and how and what should be assessed. As noted by EdCaN (2008), there is a tension between academic qualifications and a professional's competence to practise (Gibson & Soanes, 2000). Generally, there is agreement that competence assessment in nursing cannot be based only on demonstration of theoretical knowledge or technical skills but should also involve some inference about a nurse's attitudes and professional practice (EdCaN, 2008; Vernon, 2013).

The most common indicator of competence in nursing practice is demonstration of practice. However, there is considerable debate about the assessment and adequacy of performance as a valid indicator. The difficulty with measuring performance is whether demonstrating a particular skill or activity, in one area or on a particular day, indicates competence in all situations on any given day (Gibson & Soanes, 2000; Vernon, Chiarella & Papps, 2012; Vernon, 2013), and whether competence is directly observable in terms of performance of an activity (Nursing Research Unit, 2009). Research suggests that observed competent performance of tasks can only be inferred, as the measurement of underpinning competencies requires evaluation of subjective aspects such as behaviours, values, attitudes and insights that are not readily amenable to quantification (Vernon, 2013).

Numerous competence assessment tools are identified in the literature (Centre for Innovation in Professional Health Education and Research, 2007; EdCaN, 2008; Fitzgerald, Walsh & McCutcheon, 2001; Hendry, Lauder & Roxburgh, 2007; Vernon et al., 2010). In general, however, there is agreement that assessment of competence should include more than one competence indicator and assessment process (Australian Nursing and Midwifery Council, 2007; Canadian Nurses Association, 2000; EdCaN, 2008; McGrath et al., 2006; Pearson et al., 2002; Scott Tilley, 2008; Vernon, 2013), and that frameworks, standards for, and assessment of, continuing competence should relate to the individual's particular scope of practice and area of practice (Australian Nursing and Midwifery Council, 2007).

Assessment measurements outlined in CCFs are generally based on indicators such as self-assessment or direct observations by a peer, a mentor, a manager or an assessor and include some level of subjectivity (Fitzgerald, Walsh & McCutcheon, 2001; Vernon, 2013). As in any assessment process, the challenge in measuring competence and continuing competence is to ensure objectivity, validity and reliability (Vernon et al., 2010; Vernon, 2013).

In New Zealand, the Nursing Council's CCF has recently been evaluated, primarily in order to:

- explore the validity of the stipulated hours of professional development and days/hours of practice over a three-year period, as indicators of competence;
- provide information on the efficacy of undertaking a random audit of five per cent of the nursing workforce to meet recertification requirements;
- document and track the different forms of written evidence that are currently acceptable to the Nursing Council to demonstrate competence;
- identify issues related to peer assessment of competence (Vernon et al., 2010).

The outcome of this evaluation was that:

- The overwhelming consensus of key stakeholders was that the CCF is a critical and important mechanism to ensure nurses are fit and competent to practise.

● Seventy-six per cent of survey respondents believe the Nursing Council's CCF and processes for renewing practising certificates provide the mechanism to ensure nurses are competent and fit to practise.

● There is historical evidence that the development of the CCF was well researched and included extensive consultation with stakeholders (Vernon et al., 2010).

Cultural safety and cultural competence

As noted earlier, the Act requires that regulatory authorities 'set standards of clinical competence, cultural competence, and ethical conduct to be observed by health practitioners of the profession' (Health Practitioners Competence Assurance Act 2003, s 118(i)). As the Act does not define cultural competence, each regulatory authority in New Zealand has interpreted this in a different way and each has developed its own guidelines and/or statements about cultural competence. As a result varying definitions of cultural competence exist.

The Nursing Council refers to cultural safety, which is defined as:

> the effective nursing practice of a person or family from another culture, and is determined by that person or family. Culture includes, but is not restricted to, age or generation; gender; sexual orientation; occupation and socioeconomic status; ethnic origin or migrant experience; religious or spiritual belief; and disability. The nurse delivering the service will have undertaken a process of reflection on his or her own cultural identity and will recognise the impact that his or her personal culture has on his or her professional practice. Unsafe cultural practice comprises any action which diminishes, demeans or disempowers the cultural identity and wellbeing of an individual. (Nursing Council of New Zealand, 2011, p. 7)

We noted earlier that following the enactment of the Act, the Nursing Council established scopes of practice for all nursing coming under its jurisdiction. Each of these scopes of practice has competencies that each nurse must declare are met on applying for an annual practising certificate. Included in these competencies are requirements for cultural safety. We have not replicated these as they are addressed in Chapter 2. The point we make here is that nurses meet cultural competence requirements of the Act through the cultural safety competencies and associated indicators.

Historically, cultural safety was introduced into nursing to address social justice issues in relation to culture. Cultural competence was seen to be associated the dominant transcultural nursing theory of Leininger (1991, 1995, 1997) and was rejected as cultural safety was considered to be something different and unique to New Zealand (Papps, 2002a). Internationally, there is recognition that cultural safety will continue to hold value for nursing practice, research and education because of its commendation for its emphasis on critical self-reflection, critique of structures, discourses, power relations and assumptions, and because of its attachment to a social justice agenda (Browne et al., 2009).

The implementation of the cultural competence requirement of the Act by some other health regulatory authorities in New Zealand are noted briefly below. The term cultural competence is used by the Occupational Therapy Board of New Zealand; however its definition refers to culturally safe practice. The New Zealand Psychologists Board has adopted the definition of cultural safety from the guidelines of the Nursing Council. The Physiotherapy Board refers to cultural competence and defines this as '... the ability to effectively interact with and provide service to all people, demonstrating respect for diverse cultural backgrounds, values or beliefs'. The Medical Council of New Zealand ('the Medical Council') refers to cultural competence and utilises the definition provided by Durie (2001) which asserts that it refers to '... the acquisition of skills to better understand members of other cultures in order to achieve the best possible health outcome'. These definitions are available through the websites of each regulatory authority .

Hera (2013, p. 47) has provided an explanation of the Medical Council's definition of cultural competence and notes that:

> Cultural competence requires an awareness of cultural diversity and the ability to function effectively, and respectfully, when working with and treating people of different cultural backgrounds. Cultural competence means a doctor has the attitudes, skills and knowledge needed to achieve this. A culturally competent doctor will acknowledge:
>
> - that New Zealand has a culturally diverse population;
> - that a doctor's culture and belief systems influence his or her interactions with patients and accepts this may impact on the doctor patient relationship;
> - that a positive patient outcome is achieved when a doctor and patient have mutual respect and understanding.

Table 4.1 outlines examples of how some regulatory authorities have addressed cultural competence.

TABLE 4.1 *Regulatory authorities and cultural competence – key documents*

REGULATORY AUTHORITY	NAME OF DOCUMENT
Nursing Council of New Zealand	Guidelines for cultural safety in nursing
Midwifery Council of New Zealand	Statement on cultural competence
Occupational Therapy Board	Cultural competence
Physiotherapy Board	Cultural competence position statement
Medical Council of New Zealand	Statement on cultural competence
New Zealand Psychologists Board	Guidelines for cultural safety

It is recommended for further reading that the information about these regulatory authorities is accessed for full descriptions.

Cultural competence or cultural safety

In a paper about the issue of cultural competence and medical practice in New Zealand, which was presented at the Australia and New Zealand Boards and Council Conference in 2001, Durie asserted that:

> Although the differences between cultural competence and cultural safety are probably outweighed by their similarities, they have quite distinct starting points and in the New Zealand health context, somewhat different histories. Both are about the relationship between the helper and the person being helped, but cultural safety centres on the experiences of the patient, or client, while cultural competence focuses on the capacity of the health worker to improve health status by integrating culture into the clinical context. This last point is important. Recognition of culture is not by itself sufficient rationale for requiring cultural competence; instead the point of the exercise is to maximise gains from a health intervention where the parties are from different cultures. (2001, p. 2)

Cultural safety and cultural competence are different discourses. Both, however, are appropriate and neither is necessarily right or wrong. Cultural safety is about the client feeling comfortable or safe with health care, while cultural competence is about the ability of health practitioners to demonstrate what is needed to achieve that. Does it matter that there is a difference? We suggest it does not. The issue is about the competence of all health practitioners to respect cultural difference and provide competent and safe care to patients.

Demonstrating cultural competence

Practice example

As part of demonstrating that you are competent in your nursing practice, you need to provide evidence for your portfolio that relates to patient care. The issue you are most concerned about is how to obtain evidence of cultural competence.

You ask one of your colleagues, who suggests you ask some patients to write a letter to you about this.

> Identify some of the issues that arise in asking patients for written feedback.
> Write a list of the various ways of providing evidence for demonstrating competence in relation to the care you provide for patients.
> Describe some other options that may be available to you to demonstrate cultural competence.

FOR REFLECTION

Conclusion

Assessment of competence and continuing competence is fraught with a number of concerns, not least of which is what to assess and how to assess. The Nursing Council has established clearly defined competencies and indicators by which cultural safety can be assessed in both nursing education and practice. An evaluation of the Nursing Council's CCF (Vernon et al., 2010) demonstrated that the CCF it is a critical and important mechanism to ensure that nurses are fit and competent to practise and assure the public that they are safe. Many other health regulatory authorities in New Zealand have either developed or are developing frameworks to monitor the continuing competence of health practitioners who come under their jurisdiction.

> With the different definitions about cultural competence and cultural safety, what are the implications for assessment of continuing competence?
> What exactly is being assessed and how is it being assessed? How should it be assessed?
> In terms of the differences between cultural safety and cultural competence, how does a health practitioner know that the patient or client feels comfortable and/or safe?

FOR REFLECTION

References

Australian Nursing and Midwifery Council. (2007). *Development of a national framework for the demonstration of continuing competence for nurses and midwives – Literature review* (pp. 1–33). Canberra: Australian Nursing and Midwifery Council.

Browne, A. J., Varcoe, C., Smye, V., Reimer-Kirkham, S., Lyman, M. J. & Wong, S. (2009). Cultural safety and the challenges of translating critically oriented knowledge in practice. *Nursing Philosophy, 10,* 167–9.

Bryant, R. (2005). *Regulation, roles and competency development. The global nursing review initiative.* Geneva: International Council of Nurses.

Canadian Nurses Association. (2000). *A national framework for continuing competence programmes for registered nurses* (p. 32). Ottawa: Canadian Nurses Association.

Centre for Innovation in Professional Health Education and Research. (2007). *Review of work-based assessment methods.* Sydney: The University of Sydney.

Chiarella, M., Thoms, D., Lau, C. & McInnes, E. (2008). An overview of the competency movement in nursing and midwifery. *Collegian, 15*(2), 45–53.

Durie, M. (2001). Cultural competence and medical practice in New Zealand. Paper presented at Australia and New Zealand Boards and Council Conference, 22 November 2001. Retrieved 18 September 2014 from https://www.massey. ac.nz/massey/fms/Te%20Mata%20O%20Te%20Tau/Publications%20-%20 Mason/M%20Durie%20Cultural%20competence%20and%20medical%20 practice%20in%20New%20Zealand.pdf

EdCaN. (2008). *Competency assessment in nursing: A summary of literature published since 2000* (pp. 1–75). Retrieved 14 February 2014 from http//:edcan.org/pdf/ EdCancompetenciesliteraturereviewFINAL.pdf

Fitzgerald, M., Walsh, K. & McCutcheon, H. (2001). *An integrative systematic review of indicators of competence for practice and protocol for validation of indicators of competence* (pp. 1–82). Brisbane: The Queensland Nursing Council.

Gibson, F. & Soanes, L. (2000). The development of clinical competencies for use on a paediatric oncology nursing course using a nominal group technique. *Journal of Clinical Nursing, 9,* 459–69.

Goodridge, J. M. (2007). Continuing competence programmes for registered nurses: ARNNL background paper. St John's, NL: Association of Registered Nurses of Newfoundland and Labrador.

Hendry, C., Lauder, W. & Roxburgh, M. (2007). The dissemination and uptake of competency frameworks. *Journal of Research in Nursing, 12*(6), 689–700.

Hera, J. (2013). Cultural competence and patient-centred care. In I. M. St George (ed.) *Cole's Medical Practice in New Zealand* (12th edn) (pp. 44–51). Wellington: Medical Council of New Zealand.

Leininger, M. (1991). *Cultural care diversity and universality: A theory for nursing.* New York: National League for Nursing.

Leininger, M. (1995). *Transcultural nursing concepts, theories, research and practices* (2nd edn.). New York: McGraw-Hill.

Leininger, M. (1997). Transcultural nursing research to transform nursing education and practice: 40 years. *Journal of Nursing Scholarship, 29*(4), 341–7.

McGrath, P., Fox Young, S., Moxham, L., Anastasi, J., Gorman, D. & Tollefson, J. (2006). Collaborative voices: Ongoing reflections on nursing competencies. *Contemporary Nurse, 22*, 46–58.

New Zealand Government. (1997). Nurses Act 1997. Wellington: New Zealand Government.

New Zealand Government. (2003). Health Practitioners Competence Assurance Act 2003. Wellington: New Zealand Government.

Nursing Council of New Zealand. (2004). *Guidelines for professional development and recognition programmes.* Wellington: Nursing Council of New Zealand.

Nursing Council of New Zealand. (2006). *Continuing Competence Framework.* Wellington: Nursing Council of New Zealand.

Nursing Council of New Zealand. (2010a). Nursing Council of New Zealand – Definition of competence. Retrieved 27 May 2012 from http://nursingcouncil.org.nz/Nurses/Continuing-competence

Nursing Council of New Zealand. (2010b). Nursing Council of New Zealand – Definition of practising. Retrieved 9 March 2010 from http://nursingcouncil.org.nz/Nurses/Continuing-competence

Nursing Council of New Zealand. (2011). *Guidelines for cultural safety, the Treaty of Waitangi and Māori health in nursing education and practice.* Wellington: Nursing Council of New Zealand.

Nursing Council of New Zealand. (2013). *Bibliographic timeline of the introduction of cultural safety into nursing education in New Zealand 1988–2012.* Wellington: Nursing Council of New Zealand.

Nursing Research Unit. (2009). Nursing competence: What are we assessing and how should it be measured? *Policy Plus Evidence, Issues and Opinions in Healthcare, 2*(18).

Papps, E. (1997). *Knowledge and power in nursing education in New Zealand: A critical analysis of the construction of the nursing identity.* Doctor of Philosophy thesis, University of Otago, Dunedin.

Papps, E. (2002a). Cultural safety: What is the question? In E. Papps (ed.) *Nursing in New Zealand: Critical issues, different perspectives.* Auckland: Pearson Education New Zealand.

Papps, E. (2002b). *Nursing in New Zealand: Critical issues, different perspectives.* Auckland: Pearson Education New Zealand.

Papps, E. (2005). Cultural safety: Daring to be different. In D. Wepa (ed.) *Cultural safety in Aotearoa New Zealand.* Auckland: Pearson Education New Zealand.

Papps, E. & Ramsden, I. (1996). Cultural safety in nursing education: The New Zealand experience. *International Journal for Quality in Health Care, 8*(5), 491–7.

Pearson, A., Fitzgerald, M., Walsh, K. & Borbasi, S. (2002). Continuing competence and the regulation of nursing practice. *Journal of Nursing Management, 10*, 357–64.

Scott Tilley, D. D. (2008). Competency in nursing: A concept analysis. *Journal of Continuing Education in Nursing, 39*(2), 58–64.

Vernon, R. A. (2013). *Relationships between legislation, policy and continuing competence requirements for registered nurses in New Zealand.* Doctor of Philosophy thesis, University of Sydney, Sydney.

Vernon, R. (2014). Competent or just confident? *Nursing Review Series 2014, 18.*

Vernon, R., Chiarella, M. & Papps, E. (2012). New Zealand nurses' perceptions of the continuing competence framework. *International Nursing Review, 60*(1), 59–66. doi: 10.1111/inr.12001

Vernon, R., Chiarella, M. & Papps, E. (2013). Assessing the continuing competence of nurses in New Zealand. *Journal of Nursing Regulation, 3*(4), 19–24.

Vernon, R., Chiarella, M., Papps, E. & Dignam, D. (2010). *Evaluation of the continuing competence framework.* Wellington: Nursing Council of New Zealand.

Vernon, R., Chiarella, M., Papps, E. & Dignam, D. (2011). Confidence in competence: Legislation and nursing in New Zealand. *International Nursing Review, 58*(1), 103–8.

Wepa, D. (2001). An exploration of the experiences of cultural safety educators. A thesis presented in partial fulfilment of the requirements for the degree of Master of Philosophy in Social Work, Massey University, Palmerston North.

5

Culture and ethnicity WHAT IS THE QUESTION?

Dianne Wepa

Learning objectives

Having studied this chapter, you will be able to:

- know the differences in meaning between culture, race and ethnicity;

- understand the complexities of categories such as 'Pākehā', 'Māori' and 'New Zealander';

- appreciate the future positioning of your own practice within the contexts of monoculturalism, biculturalism and multiculturalism.

Key terms and concepts

- culture

- descent

- ethnicity

- Māori

- monoculturalism

- multiculturalism

- New Zealander

- Pākehā

- race

- self-identity

- sprituality

Introduction

The common catch-phrase 'Culture! We don't have a culture!' is often the reply to the question: 'What is your culture?' when it is posed to New Zealanders today. Since the implementation of cultural safety in the schools of nursing and midwifery, students have been introduced to concepts that were not as evident in most programmes prior to the early 1990s. Topics such as culture and the dynamics of power are now commonplace within these programmes. Similarly, with the movement towards 'doing with' as opposed to 'doing for' the client, students are required to possess an awareness of their values, beliefs, biases and prejudices. The first step towards cultural safety, therefore, is for a person to have sufficient awareness of their own culture.

So, for many students who ascribe to the dominant culture and values in Aoteroa New Zealand, they may well ask the question: 'Why do I need to learn about my culture?' This is particularly difficult for students to reflect on if they believe that they are just 'normal' and culture is something Māori or immigrants possess. The short answer is that once there is clarity about people's own values and beliefs (which are key components of culture) and how they affect their living, then they are in a better position to appreciate that other people do things differently. Nurses and midwives work with people from a range of cultures and circumstances. To be effective, therefore, they must become aware of their own culture and the impact this has on their practice. Nurses and midwives can unknowingly place other people's cultural perspectives at risk. This is exhibited when people avoid going to a health service because they perceive the health professional to be disrespectful of their cultural practices and traditions.

This chapter assists the journey of nursing people from cultures other than one's own. Misconceptions surrounding culture and ethnicity are clarified with a view to providing a common understanding of individual and sociological notions of culture, race, ethnicity, self-identity, monoculturalism, biculturalism, multiracial, multiculturalism, interculturalism and super-diversity in relation to nursing and midwifery practice.

Culture

There are various definitions available to describe 'culture'. During my teaching career within the field of cultural safety, I developed the following definition:

> Our way of living is our culture. It's our taken-for-grantedness that determines and defines our culture. The way we brush our teeth, the way we bury people, the way we express ourselves through our art, religion, eating habits, rituals, humour, science, law, and sport; the way we celebrate occasions (from 21sts, to weddings, to birthdays) is our culture. All these actions we carry out consciously and unconsciously.

Broadly speaking, culture includes our activities, ideas, our belongings, relationships, what we do, say, think, are. Culture is central to the manner in which all people develop and grow and how they view themselves and others. It is the outcome of the influences and principles of people's ancestors, ideology, philosophies of life and geographical situation. A culture is never completely static and all cultures are affected and modified by the proximity and influences of other cultures.

Similarities between all cultures

When discussing culture, I find it useful to include key aspects that everyone has in common. Within the context of health care, professionals can only be influenced by someone if they are willing to relate with them. With this in mind, there may be a way in which a professional and the client can work with shared values, beliefs, traditions, and experiences.

Here are some generalisations about all cultures that you may want to discuss in small groups. What examples for each statement exist in your culture?

> All cultures face life, birth and death.
> All cultures are concerned with survival.
> All cultures are concerned with interpreting the universe.
> All cultures have rules structuring social relationships.
> All cultures are concerned with perpetuating their culture.
> All cultures use language as a means of transmitting information from one generation to another.

Material and non-material culture

According to Giddens and Sutton (2013), there are two key components to culture. They are material and non-material culture. Non-material culture consists of the words people use, the ideas, customs and beliefs they hold and the habits they follow. Material culture consists of objects made by people such as cars, mobile phones, buildings, ditches, cultivated farms – in fact, any physical substance that has been changed and used by people. Material culture is the result of non-material culture. Without non-material culture, the material culture is meaningless.

In modern-day culture, physical artifacts such as mobile phones have cultural meanings for the people who produce and use them. A mobile phone is not simply a phone to call someone. Mobile phones have meaning in terms of non-material culture ranging from the type of phone someone owns through to its functions. The type or brand of phone may tell us the meaning ascribed to the phone as opposed to its purpose or function.

Demonstrating material and non-material culture

Practice example 1

One day my friend lost her mobile phone. The phone was expensive and was manufactured by a well-known producer of mobile phones. It had a large touch screen and came with a special bag that protected the cover of the phone and also housed all her identification, coffee cards and cash-flow cards. These were a few elements of material culture associated with the phone. The non-material aspects of the phone were my friend's contacts saved in the phone, the phone's ability to connect to social media, emails and a myriad of other functions that I couldn't understand. My friend was very upset that she had lost her phone. My reply to her was 'You can always get another phone and cards'. My friend became more upset with my response to her phone being lost.

FOR REFLECTION

> What was more important to my friend in this situation – non-material or material culture?
> How might this situation be related to a clinical setting?

Race and 'isms'

A term that is diametrically opposed to culture is 'race'. Race cannot be defined with any accuracy. Generally speaking, the concept of race assumes that the phenotype (or physical characteristics) is an appropriate way of classifying people into social groups. Furthermore, the difference in phenotype becomes synonymous with variations in intellect and abilities. It assumes that people who share a phenotype will act in a certain way. From this basis it becomes possible to 'rank' races according to their superiority and inferiority (Miles, 1989).

From a sociological and political viewpoint, the idea of 'race' is problematic. It originated during European colonisation in the 18th and 19th centuries. Classification of people according to their appearance helped Europeans make sense of human diversity (Fleras & Spoonley, 1999). It became part of the ideological justification for colonial exploitation, as it assisted the practice of slavery and eugenics (the notion that populations could be improved by using knowledge about genetics). In 1975 the United Nations refuted the notion that some races were superior and others inferior and called for an end to the reductionist method of measuring people's identity in 'drops of blood'.

The primary problem with the idea of race is that it is an arbitrary form of social classification. Physical difference is an obvious and easily employed means of classifying people. Its use remains a way of explaining the social world that is supported by major agencies such as the police or media that report events. Such agencies often use the term without critique, thus perpetuating the view that race is important. For example, television shows such as *Police Ten-7* have been criticised for portraying Māori and Pacific people in a negative light (Podvoiskis, 2012). The predominantly Pākehā police officers are seen arresting mostly Māori and Pacific people for committing traditional 'street' crimes such as drug and antisocial offending, and violence, while under-representing other common 'white-collar' offences such as fraud.

The resulting behaviours demonstrated against groups of people based on their race are termed 'monoculturalism' and 'ethnocentrism'. Monoculturalism exists when the dominant culture controls all the major institutions and restricts expression of others' culture (Giddens & Sutton, 2013). In a healthcare context an institutional policy that restricts visitors within a ward to 'immediate family only' is an example of monoculturalism. In this instance, the 'nuclear' definition of 'family' views mum, dad and kids as the acceptable version, thereby negating other variations such as whānau and same-sex couples. On a personal level, the practice of ethnocentrism can flourish under a monocultural regime. Ethnocentrism is the belief that your own cultural background, including ways of analysing problems, values, beliefs, language, and verbal and non-verbal communication, is the correct one (Chaney & Martin, 2011). An example within health care is the belief that the correct method of nourishment for an infant consists of 'four-hourly feeds' despite a new mother's request to feed on demand. Many ethnocentric views within health care stem from the nursing and midwifery context where traditional ways of treating people become common practice. If new mothers were asked why they required to feed their babies every four hours, the reply might be 'because we've always done it that way'. This response is couched within the concepts of 'tradition' and 'practice'. In this context, tradition is about how nurses and midwives were traditionally taught to implement four-hourly feeds regardless of the requirements of the mother and baby. Practice relates to carrying out the practice of four-hourly feeds to the level expected by the hospital.

Ethnicity

I have developed my own definition for 'ethnicity' as follows:

> refers to the cultural practices and outlooks of a community which identifies
> them as a distinctive social group. Cultural practices include festivals,
> rituals and celebrations. Outlooks include a commonly held view of the
> world through religion, spirituality or shared historical events such as war
> or migration.

Ethnicity does not have the connotations of 'race' as it is based on more factors than physical characteristics, nor does it require a dominant group to label
other groups. Members of an ethnic group:

- share a sense of common origins;
- claim a common and distinctive history or common destiny;
- possess one or more dimensions of a collective cultural identity, for example, language, physical appearance;
- feel a sense of unique collective solidarity.

Several factors serve to differentiate between ethnic groups. They include:

- language;
- religion;
- history;
- styles of dress;
- ancestry;
- adornment.

Everyone belongs to a variety of groups (for example, church, sport, leisure
organisations). Ethnicity is one further dimension of such group identity. It
captures the sense of belonging which, in turn, helps mould an identity for an
individual (McLennan, Ryan & Spoonley, 2004). The 'self-identification' of a
person with an ethnic group can be:

- influenced by social and political factors;
- inconsistent over time as one group merges into another;
- difficult if there are a number of identities.

'Descent' from a particular ethnic group is now used in the collection of statistics. Most reasons for collecting statistics on ethnicity are political. Three
explanations exist to support this view. First, for most of New Zealand's history, the biological concept of race was used to progress policies of assimilation.

For example, the Māori Affairs Act 1953 defined someone as Māori if they possessed half or more Māori blood. The desire by the government to calculate Māori numbers assisted policies such as 'pepper-potting' where the method of dispersing Māori houses amongst European houses promoted closer integration and reduced the continuation of tribal practices (Durie, 1998).

The second political reason for collecting statistics related to immigration. Categories assisted with immigration of settlers from Europe, the Pacific and, more recently, Asia. As New Zealand's first immigration document, Te Tiriti o Waitangi/the Treaty of Waitangi, signed in 1840, encouraged safe settlement for people from Britain. After World War II, assisted and unrestricted immigration was extended to people from selected Western European countries and other New Zealand territories such as the Cook Islands, Niue and Tokelau (Spoonley, Pearson & Macpherson, 1996).

The third reason is the need to plan for social equity. The combination of ethnicity data, vital statistics (births, death, marriages) and the census provides a complete picture of the situation of the population of New Zealand today. The move towards cultural affiliation and self-identification as part of this process aims to reduce the stigma attached to identity. It also aims to promote measures that reduce a range of inequities within the major social indicators of society (such as health, housing, justice and welfare).

Māori

Prior to European contact, Māori had no single term for themselves. People were distinguished from one another by their tribal names. The word 'Māori' means 'normal', 'usual' or 'ordinary' and, through usage, has become capitalised to refer to the Māori people collectively.

Māori identity and well-being has become the focus of a government-led project called Te Kupenga. Health statistics have traditionally considered negative information on Māori health and well-being. Te Kupenga provides an overall picture of the social, cultural, and economic well-being of Māori in New Zealand. It contains general social and economic well-being measures, and also introduced new measures based on the Māori perspective of well-being. Four areas of cultural well-being noted are:

- wairua (spirituality);
- tikanga (Māori customs and practices);
- te reo Māori (the Māori language);
- whanaungatanga (social connectedness).

Results from Te Kupenga, and conducted by Statistics New Zealand, noted that 70 per cent of Māori adults said it was important for them to be involved with Māori culture. Fifty-five per cent had some ability to speak te reo Māori, and 83 per cent said their whānau were doing well or extremely well (Statistics New Zealand, 2014). Te Kupenga will become an ongoing survey and needs to be considered when reviewing other health statistics about Māori.

FOR REFLECTION

Consider the four areas of well-being identified in Te Kupenga. What four areas could be applied to your culture?

Pākehā

Like many other countries outside Europe, Aotearoa New Zealand has a recent history of being colonised by the British. In this country there is a special word for the European-originated culture – Pākehā. Bolstad reflects on this term:

> What I like about the word *Pākehā* is that it reminds me that I am a New Zealander, not a European. It was developed at a time of friendship between European explorers and Māori. (2004, p.16)

With the publication of Michael King's book *Being Pākehā* (1985) came questions of identity in the late 1980s and 1990s. The term became a marker of difference *from* Europeans as well as a relationship *with* Māori. As the dominant group, however, Pākehā may view their culture as the national culture. The irony here is that the national culture is often portrayed in terms of Māori cultural icons such as the koru or the haka. In this sense, Pākehā culture may be the national culture in terms of providing the pervasive, common sense underpinnings for the ordering of social life, but Māori culture is the national culture when distinctiveness and ethnic exoticism is called for (Spoonley, Pearson & Macpherson, 1996). Pākehā could therefore be referred to as an ethnic category (a group of people sharing identifiable characteristics such as those already mentioned) but has not yet achieved the status of an 'ethnic community'. An ethnic community emphasises a sense of group consciousness or sense of group belonging and solidarity. This is often achieved where a group is a cultural minority and has experienced oppression as a minority (Spoonley, Pearson & Macpherson, 1996). Majority groups generally do not have these experiences. The exception would include overseas travel where Pākehā may discover that they do indeed have a culture which is to be celebrated as unique and of value.

As the second indigenous culture in New Zealand, Pākehā culture could claim 'indigeneity' because it does not exist anywhere else in the world.

> What terms do you feel comfortable using to identify your ethnicity?
> People tend to identify themselves as New Zealanders when they travel outside of New Zealand. What might you think contributes to this change in identity from living within and outside of New Zealand?

We are all New Zealanders

National identities evolve over time. New Zealand identity has changed due to the shifting relationship with the United Kingdom, changing relationships among Māori, Pākehā and newer New Zealanders, and the interaction of New Zealand with other countries and cultures. Defining a national identity is not simple. While people may describe themselves as 'New Zealanders', how they define their 'New Zealand-ness' will vary from person to person. For example, some people might see their New Zealand identity in terms of history or achievements in sports, arts or other endeavours, while others might use national symbols and icons.

Phrases like 'we are all New Zealanders' or 'we are all one people' are sometimes used as a rationale for maintaining Pākehā dominance and undermining Māori as the indigenous group within New Zealand (Callister, 2004). There is debate about the use of the term 'New Zealander' as the New Zealand Census has recorded 'New Zealander' since 2001. In 2006, 11 per cent of the population identified themselves as a New Zealander and the responses counted as 'European' were moved into a new group called 'other ethnicities' (Callister, Didham & Kivi, 2009). One problem with the creation of this category is that it becomes difficult to predict population growth in terms of births and deaths.

If all people chose New Zealander as a category on statistical information then policy and funding of social areas that affect the country may not be as accurate as previously encountered. What do you think would be a solution to this issue?

Biculturalism

In 1986 the New Zealand Government's Department of Social Welfare published *Puao Te Ata Tu: Daybreak, the Ministerial Advisory Committee on a Māori Perspective for the Department of Social Welfare*. This document challenged the racism that existed in government departments and provided the catalyst for the introduction of 'biculturalism' education for all state employees.

Simply put, biculturalism is the coexistence of two distinct cultures. Durie offers the following definition:

> Biculturalism exists when the values and traditions of both cultures are reflected in society's customs, laws, practices, and institutional arrangements, and with both cultures sharing control over resources and decision making. (1998, p. 101)

Cooney's definition relates specifically to nursing:

> Biculturalism is a significant concept in New Zealand since, by accepting that we are a bicultural country, it ensures that Māori are given rightful recognition as the indigenous people and therefore obligations under the Treaty must be addressed. Cultural safety places considerable emphasis on this bicultural relationship. (1994, p. 9)

Durie (1998) believes that biculturalism needs to be considered as a continuum with a range of goals, from understanding Māori health issues on a practice level, through to formal joint ventures between Māori and the Crown. Within the cultural safety process, biculturalism firmly positions Māori as partners with the Crown (and its agencies). The experiences of both these parties in the 19th and 20th centuries have also grounded nurses and midwives as responsive agents of change. In the 21st century, the foundation concepts learnt from the bicultural relationship have placed nurses and midwives in a strong position to accept new challenges within other environments. On a personal level, nurses and midwives are continuously engaging in bicultural encounters, for example, there is always one giver of the message (nurse/midwife) and receiver of the message regardless of the number of people listening. I could have one patient or whānau receiving the message or a whole room of people. They are all engaging in a bicultural encounter as each individual will receive the message through their own cultural frameworks.

Multiculturalism

As New Zealand has become increasingly multiracial, there has been a move by the government from assimilation towards acceptance of cultural diversity. Such a view implies a degree of sensitivity to migrants in particular. The specific health needs of New Zealand's rapidly growing migrant communities can be complex as the 2013 Census revealed that people of Asian, Middle Eastern,

Latin American, African and other descent now comprise nearly 15 per cent of the population compared with Pacific (7.4%) and Māori (15%) (Spoonley, 2014).

Within a cultural safety framework, the intention is not to attempt to know about all these cultures and their nuances. The focus, therefore, is to be authentic as a nurse or midwife, and to support people to practise their cultural traditions within a healthcare setting. Practices may include prayers and hymns, special food, speaking a different language, and involvement of the wider family unit in daily cares. To demonstrate multiculturalism, therefore, involves having a strong sense of self which includes knowing your own culture, traditions, biases and taken-for-grantedness. Self-reflective practice is also crucial so that the health professionals can self-manage their behaviour especially if they notice that they begin to prevent people from continuing with their cultural practices while they are receiving a healthcare service from them.

A personal reflection by William Pua

Practice example 2

A Samoan colleague shared a personal experience where there was a missed opportunity to implement cultural safety with his aiga or family. Consider the areas that could have been addressed to provide a better outcome for all parties in this extract.

I was born in Grey Lynn in the 1960s. My parents came from Samoa, in search of a better life. There were six of us. My dad was a matai or chief in Samoa and a teacher but his qualifications were not recognised so he worked for the post office in the mailroom sorting mail. My mum worked as a sewing machinist and after that job she also worked as a cleaner in the evening. We took turns to help Mum with her cleaning. Mum developed diabetes, and with this she had cataracts, which caused her to be blind and over time she had renal problems, which made her very sickly. My dad became sick as well. I remember the day that my dad woke up from a nap. He was talking but we couldn't understand what he was saying. He was speaking gibberish, nothing made sense. I was so scared. I didn't know what a stroke was but I could see the fear in my dad's eyes. Three hours earlier, he had gone to have a nap...then he woke up and wasn't able to speak. We just panicked and didn't know what to do. Later on we were told that he had had a stroke and that it had affected his ability to speak any language at all as my dad was bilingual (he spoke Samoan and English). Strangely enough, despite this proclamation, our dad still had the ability to speak in Samoan. Whilst it was stilted and laboured, he was still able to communicate. However, he could no longer speak English – that language was seemingly lost.

When the physiotherapist came to visit Dad, we were alarmed by the rude tone adopted. I remember thinking 'This is no way a health professional or anyone for that matter should speak to my dad, let alone a matai or chief'. The physio was frustrated by

Dad's lack of progress and the lack of commitment to doing his exercises. When the physio would talk to Dad, it was hard for us to listen. I had never heard my dad being spoken to in such a rude manner. We rallied around Dad, to protect him from this rude person. I wished we had understood what the physio was trying to do and that he had understood how we would interpret his approach.

In the end, I regret that our dad did not get the rehabilitation care that he needed. To me, the notion of cultural safety needs to incorporate a health approach which embraces and understands the cultural worlds, beliefs and values that patients and their aiga/families bring with them. If this had happened, the healthcare professionals would have known why we were responding in this protective manner as a direct result of the inappropriate approach, and would have worked with us as a family and enlisted us to support their work plan.

Culture and spirituality

Spirituality is increasingly considered to be a contributing factor towards a person's health and well-being within New Zealand. The term spirituality can be confusing at times as it can be misinterpreted to mean religion. I have defined spirituality as 'a focus on a spiritual world that develops within a person and can be considered private'. Religion can be defined as belief in god or gods that are worshipped through rituals, a specific belief system, code of conduct, symbols and worship'.

During colonisation, missionaries introduced Christianity as a religion to Māori. Many Māori chiefs encouraged their people to convert to Christianity as the missionaries were viewed as men of God with a strong sense of spirituality or wairua which Māori valued. Today Māori are still considered to be connected to their spirituality, so much so that illness can prevail in some instances if this connection is not maintained. The four-sided house or 'te whare tapa wha' coined by Durie (1998) depicts the key components that support health for Māori – taha whānau (family well-being), taha hinengaro (cognitive and emotional well-being), taha tinana (physical well-being), and taha wairua (spiritual well-being). According to Durie (1998) if each taha, or side of the house, is not supported then the person may become unwell. Many health professionals have become familiar with te whare tapa wha and are encouraged to consider each aspect of this framework when engaging with Māori.

Within a biomedical setting, such as a medical or surgical ward, the physical well-being of a patient has traditionally taken priority. Within nursing and midwifery the curing/caring dynamic is a constant challenge. Curing can easily take precedence over the caring as a patient becomes anonymous and categorised as a condition. Utilising te whare tapa wha supports the rebalance of caring where patients are free to express their spirituality within health care. Such an expression is increasingly commonplace during birth and the stages within end-of-life. Reflecting on your own views is a starting point to help support others when spirituality or religion is foremost in people's minds.

Spirituality within health care can be a sensitive issue to deal with especially during times of stress. The actions that health professionals take can either hinder or enhance the experience for patients that are unfamiliar with the biomedical setting. Providing the opportunity for patients to express their spirituality or religion can also bring healing and closure for all.

> On what occasions do you think you would need to consider spirituality or religion in health care?
> How might you respond to a situation where you did not agree with someone practising their spirituality or religion in health care?
> What actions could you take to support someone requiring spiritual or religious support?

FOR REFLECTION

Conclusion

This chapter has provided an understanding of common terms and concepts that are frequently discussed within cultural safety education. Misconceptions surrounding culture, ethnicity and spirituality in New Zealand have been challenged and debated so that clarity can be achieved on what is still considered an evolving topic. With the effects of globalisation, increasing migration and the reassertion of indigenous rights, the 21st century holds complex and varied challenges for nurses and midwives. The implementation of multiculturalism need not be at odds with biculturalism as long as Māori are recognised as equal partners with the Crown rather than having to compete for cultural space with other cultures. Once biculturalism becomes normalised within nursing and midwifery, multiculturalism will unfold thereafter. Whether you position yourself within any of these paradigms, in the final analysis, possessing an awareness of one's own place in the world together with power sharing will create a culturally safe workplace for ourselves and the people we serve.

References

Bolstad, R. (2004). *Transforming communication: Leading-edge professional and personal skills* (2nd edn.). Auckland: Pearson Education New Zealand.

Callister, P. (2004). Seeking an ethnic identity: Is 'New Zealander' a valid ethnic category? *New Zealand Population Review, 30*(1&2), 5–22.

Callister, P., Didham, R. & Kivi, A. (2009). Who are we? The conceptualisation and expression of ethnicity. *Official Statistics Research Series, 4.*

Chaney, L. & Martin, J. (2011). *Intercultural business communication.* New Jersey: Prentice Hall.

Cooney, C. (1994). A comparative analysis of transcultural nursing and cultural safety. *Nursing Praxis in New Zealand, 9,* 6–12.

Department of Social Welfare. (1986). *Puao Te Ata Tu: Daybreak, the Ministerial Advisory Committee on a Māori perspective for the Department of Social Welfare.* Wellington: Department of Social Welfare.

Durie, M. (1998). *Whaiora: Māori health development* (2nd edn.). Auckland: Oxford University Press.

Fleras, A. & Spoonley, P. (1999). *Recalling Aotearoa: Indigenous politics and ethnic relations in New Zealand.* Auckland: Oxford University Press.

Giddens, A. & Sutton, P. W. (2013). *Sociology* (7th edn.). Oxford: Polity Press.

King, M. (1985). *Being Pākehā.* Auckland: Hodder and Stoughton.

McLennan, G., Ryan, A. & Spoonley, P. (2004). *Exploring society: Sociology for New Zealand students* (2nd edn.). Auckland: Pearson Education New Zealand.

Miles, R. (1989). *Racism.* London: Routledge.

Podvoiskis, G. M. (2012). Reel cops: Exploring the representation of policing on *Police Ten 7.* Unpublished Master of Arts in Criminology, Victoria University of Wellington, Wellington.

Spoonley, P. (2014). Census 2013. More ethnicities than the world's countries. *New Zealand Herald,* 11 December.

Spoonley, P., Pearson, D. & Macpherson, C. (eds). (1996). *Nga Patai: Racism and ethnic relations in Aotearoa/New Zealand.* Palmerston North: Dunmore.

Statistics New Zealand. (2014). Te Kupenga 2013. Wellington.

6

Te Tiriti o Waitangi/ Treaty of Waitangi 1840 ITS INFLUENCE ON HEALTH PRACTICE

Denise Wilson and Riripeti Haretuku

Learning objectives

Having studied this chapter, you will be able to:

- explain key influences leading up to the signing of the Te Tiriti o Waitangi/Treaty of Waitangi;

- understand the impact that the Te Tiriti o Waitangi/Treaty of Waitangi had post-1840 on Māori health and health practice in early Aotearoa New Zealand;

- understand the relevance of Te Tiriti o Waitangi/Treaty of Waitangi today in the context of Māori health disparities;

- understand how Te Tiriti o Waitangi/Treaty of Waitangi applies to you as a health practitioner in New Zealand.

Key terms and concepts

- biculturalism (partnership relationship with Māori)

- Kāwanatanga (governorship)

- mana (authority and status)

- taonga (land, estates, forests, taonga (health))

- tino rangatiratanga (sovereignty)

- Te Tiriti o Waitangi (Treaty of Waitangi)

- tangata whenua (indigenous)

Introduction

In the 1800s New Zealand was a very different country to the British colony that emerged after February 1840. Although the Māori world was changing, a decade before the signing of the Treaty of Waitangi ('the Treaty') Māori retained their autonomy. At this time it was estimated that the Māori population was approximately 150 000 (Kingi, 2005). Pre-1830 Māori were a vibrant and healthy people. They were international traders within and outside of New Zealand, with their own bank. They had total guardianship of their 66 million acres, resources and other assets.

During the 1830s resident Europeans, however, were few – about 1400 in the North Island and 500 in the South Island. With increasing European settlement came the introduction of arms and what was known as the musket wars resulting in notable decreases in the populations of some iwi. Traders and settlers exploited resources, and while some missionaries and traders purchased smaller pieces of land, speculators acquired large amounts of land. Furthermore, missionaries introduced Christian beliefs and practices (Orange, 2004).

Nonetheless, in direct contrast to promising developments associated with international trade, the health of Māori visibly declined due to the harmful impacts of introduced diseases, warfare and social change. In addition to declining health, Māori had increasing concerns about the lawlessness of settlers in Aotearoa New Zealand. This led to Māori leaders petitioning the British Government to address this matter. In 1832 James Busby was appointed the British 'Resident' in New Zealand, responsible for the law and order of British subjects, backed by periodic visits from a warship from Sydney Royal Navy squadron. Busby also encouraged Māori chiefs to organise themselves into an entity more recognisable to the British Government to make and enforce British style 'laws' (Orange, 2004). This approach was unusual, as in some countries that the British migrated to, the indigenous people were almost ignored or brushed aside because they lacked the military and social organisation to resist settlement (Sinclair, 1980).

In 1835 the need for a declaration of independence appears to have been triggered by a Frenchman, Baron De Thierry, who claimed that he would set up a 'sovereign and independent state' in the Hokianga District. Busby saw this as an opportunity for Māori chiefs to set up a 'government', something he had been directed to do among Māori. The Declaration of Independence was drafted by Busby, the missionary Henry Williams and the mission printer William Colenso and signed by 52 chiefs (Appendix 1). Busby believed the Declaration of Independence would inhibit other countries from making agreements with Māori chiefs (State Services Commission, 2005). In 1836 the British Government, through the House of Commons, ratified the Declaration of Independence 1835 and acknowledged the Confederation title and Māori sovereignty as indisputable (Confederation of Chiefs of the United Tribes of Aotearoa, 2010). Nevertheless, Busby's anticipation of Māori chiefs forming a government did not eventuate (Orange, 2004).

Here are the key points of the Declaration of Independence:

- is an international declaration;
- recognises the sovereignty of the independent iwi (tribes) of New Zealand;
- was signed on 28 October 1835;
- was witnessed by Crown residents;
- was the forerunner to the Treaty of Waitangi;
- has a flag to symbolise tribal rights to trade as independent nations;
- has been disregarded by New Zealand governments and the education system.

Ongoing concerns existed about settlers' and traders' unruly behaviours, declining Māori health and the negative impacts on Māori. Britain's colonisation of New Zealand included regulation of not only British subjects' unruly behaviours but also the purchasing of land (Mutu, 2010). Transactions for the purchasing of land from Māori were carried out in unfair and unjust ways, and increasingly left Māori more and more disadvantaged. In 1839, the British Government appointed William Hobson to acquire sovereignty over New Zealand. On the 5 February 1840, Hobson and Busby met with a confederation of chiefs at Waitangi and a draft of the Treaty in English (Appendix 2) was prepared that Henry Williams undertook to translate into te reo Māori, known as Te Tiriti o Waitangi.

On 6 February 1840 the Treaty was signed by William Hobson (as the agent of the British Crown) and hapū Māori at Waitangi in the Bay of Islands, North Island, New Zealand. Although many chiefs were suspicious at the time, approximately 40 chiefs signed (Kingi, 2005; Orange, 2004). Thereafter, copies of the Treaty were taken to various points around the New Zealand, leading to approximately 540 chiefs signing the Māori text by September of 1840 (Appendix 2), although not all chiefs signed this document.

Kingi (2007) states that the purpose of the Treaty was to 'protect and promote Māori health', however its prominence and place in health has been dependent upon the political will of successive governments. It is against this backdrop that a number of issues, and subsequent causes of contention, arose from the Treaty's content. These issues included:

- The English version of the Treaty bore little resemblance to the Māori language version Māori chiefs signed (Mutu, 2010).
- Britain's view was that the Treaty applied to all Māori despite some chiefs not signing.
- Britain's view was that Māori were not a sovereign nation (Kingi, 2005).

- British and Māori interpretations differed, creating problems in its application (see Table 6.1).
- Confusion caused long-term breaches, the confiscation and unethical seizure of Māori land by the Crown, and the enactment of legislation and policies that aimed to further disadvantage Māori (Moon, 2007).

Mulholland and Tawhai stated:

> The 6th of February 1840 marked a downward spiral for Māori, a loss of political autonomy that would result in the tangata whenua being culturally, socially and economically bereft in their own lands. (2010, p. 1)

Despite international rule of *contra proferentem* that the indigenous language version should be upheld when treaties have been drafted in English, for instance, it is the English version that is considered the official version.

TABLE 6.1 *Interpretations of the English and Māori texts of Te Tiriti o Waitangi/Treaty of Waitangi*

TREATY INTENT AND ARTICLES	TREATY OF WAITANGI ENGLISH VERSION	TE TIRITI O WAITANGI TRANSLATION OF THE MĀORI VERSION SIGNED BY APPROXIMATELY 540 MĀORI CHIEFS
Preamble	A response to growing numbers of settlers coming to New Zealand.	About protecting Māori, given the lawlessness of settlers.
	Queen Victoria's desire was to protect the rights and property of Māori, ensure peace and establish a government to keep law and order.	Queen Victoria's desire was to preserve Māori chieftainship over lands and to keep peace and order by establishing government.
	William Hobson was appointed to act on Queen Victoria's behalf.	William Hobson was appointed to act on Queen Victoria's behalf.
Article 1	Māori Chiefs of Confederation of United Tribes of New Zealand and separate and independent chiefs, **gave up** their authority and rights of **sovereignty** 'absolutely and without reservation'.	Māori **gave governorship** of their land to the Queen.
Article 2	**Guaranteed** Māori **'full, exclusive and undisturbed possession'** of their land. Māori gave the Queen the exclusive right to buy their lands.	**Guaranteed** Māori **protection** and affirmed their right of **tino rangatiratanga** (authority and self-determination) over their lands, villages and precious possessions. Māori agreed to sell land to the Queen at an agreed price, if willing.
Article 3	**Guaranteed protection** of all 'natives of New Zealand'. Māori afforded the **'rights and privileges'** of 'British subjects'.	Guaranteed Māori **protection and the same rights** as the people of Britain.

Māori health and Te Tiriti o Waitangi/Treaty of Waitangi 1840–1986

As early as 1837, Busby became concerned about the declining health of Māori associated with the ad hoc approach to colonisation and noted, in particular, the need for British intervention (Kingi, 2005). High rates of Māori mortality resulted from musket warfare, starvation, and an absence of immunity to diseases and epidemics introduced by European settlers. Furthermore, in response to Britian's colonising agenda, Māori endured significant land loss together with social and economic changes that disrupted their social cohesion (Lange, 1999). After the signing of the Treaty, and despite much attention paid to Māori being a 'dying race', the government and health sector overlooked their Treaty obligations and the need to resolve the poor status of Māori health (Lange, 1999).

Western-based health care for Māori was disorganised, compromised by funding constraints and was largely provided by missionaries who only offered rudimentary care. Dow (1999) claimed this '... helped shape the reaction of Māori [sic] to Western medicine' (p. 18). Māori health status was also compromised by the limited efficacy of Western medicine at that time. A mistaken belief emerged that Māori were a 'dying race' due to their rampant depopulation because of infectious disease epidemics (such as smallpox and cholera), accompanied by ongoing debates about the funding of health services for Māori. Nevertheless, halting this predicted extinction of Māori appeared to be related to the introduction of a rudimentary vaccination programme rather than the availability of effective health services (Dow, 1999).

Article 3 of the Treaty set out Māori rights to protection, and access to the same quality of health and standard of living as British citizens. Despite this stated intention, the Māori population steadily declined from approximately 150 000 in the early 1800s to 37 500 by the time of the 1871 census. Reid and Robson (2006) assert that 'The story of Māori health is one of systematic disparities in health outcomes ...' (p. 17). Cultural identity and connectedness was negatively impacted for many Māori through their dispossession of land, loss of language and traditional cultural practices, and restricted access to social and cultural resources resulting from urbanisation policies (Ihimaera, 1998). These issues were further compounded by numerous detrimental policy and legislative decisions over time, such as the restriction of Māori identity by blood quantum.

For many years only those with 50 per cent or more 'Māori blood' were officially recognised as Māori (Hunn, 1960) – a state that continued until 1986.

Historical and ongoing contemporary traumas have influenced the health and well-being of Māori, confirmed by the significant health inequities Māori experience, such as major diseases (like cardiovascular disease, cancer and diabetes) and the consequent premature mortalities, infectious diseases, suicides and incidences of self-harm, mental illnesses, and accidental injuries (Reid & Robson, 2006). Furthermore, Māori remain subjected to inequities in access to health resources, access to health services and the quality of care needed to reduce health inequities.

Does the Treaty impact the health of Māori today? Explain the rationale for your response.

Variable government responsiveness

The first New Zealand Parliament, set up under the Constitution Act 1852, excluded Māori. Governor Grey argued that native [electoral] districts were not needed since the 'amalgamation of races' (or the creation of 'one people') was proceeding well. In 1864, Māori land was confiscated in Taranaki, Waikato, Tauranga, Eastern Bay of Plenty and Māhaka-Waikare under the New Zealand Settlements Act. This confiscation had detrimental effects on the health and well-being of Māori living in these areas, evident in their Treaty of Waitangi tribunal claims.

Under the Māori Representation Act 1867, four Māori seats were established and remained unchanged until 1996 when mixed member proportional representation was introduced. In 1877, the Treaty was judged as having neither judicial nor constitutional roles in government on the basis that Māori were 'savages' and therefore incapable of signing the Treaty (State Services Commission, 2005). Furthermore, voting rights were contingent on individual land ownership, contrary to the collective guardianship approach to land by Māori.

By the 1900s, Māori participation in health care became evident, albeit constrained by legislation, health policies, professional and institutional domination, and insufficient funding (Durie, 1998; 2001). During this time Māori leaders, such as Maui Pomare, Te Rangihiroa and Te Puea Herangi, advocated for improvements in Māori health. In 1937 the Women's Health League, Te Rōpū o Te Ora, was formed under the guidance of nurse R.T. Cameron.

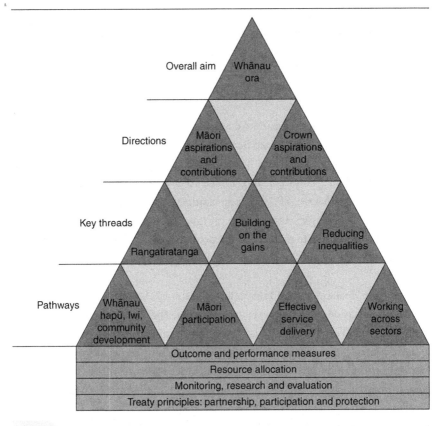

FIGURE
6.1
He Korowai Oranga framework – the Māori Health Strategy
Source: New Zealand Ministry of Health (2014)

Te Rōpū Wāhine Māori Toko i te Ora (the Māori Women's Welfare League) was established in the 1940s and led by Dame Whina Cooper, who focused on promoting healthy whānau and improving housing, health and education for Māori. In the 1970s and 1980s, Māori vocalised their dissatisfaction with the ongoing inequalities and inequities Māori were experiencing in health, education and social areas.

While gains have been made in Māoi health since the 1980s, disparities and inequities remain and, up until the early 2000s, the role of the Treaty has waxed and waned dependent upon the political environment. He Korowai Oranga – the Māori Health Strategy (King & Turia, 2002) is an example of the Treaty being implemented with Māori and the government negotiating whānau ora (whānau well-being) as an overall goal (Figure 6.1). This has been updated so pae ora (healthy futures) is now the overall aim, achieved through whānau ora, mauri ora (healthy individuals) and wai ora (healthy environments) (Ministry of Health, 2014).

Legislation

In 1907 the Tohunga Suppression Act was passed facilitating the government's desire to establish Western-based health care in New Zealand. This legislation prohibited Tohunga (traditional Māori healers) from practising and was not repealed until 1962. Tohunga were forced to covertly practice resulting in a loss of knowledge (Moon, 2003). Moon claims this legislation '... brutally cut a swathe through many Māori communities, and was instrumental in forcing those communities to shift from a dependence on traditional methods and ideas about healing and knowledge to solely contemporary Western models' (p. 10).

The New Zealand Public Health and Disability Act 2000 is the first piece of health legislation to incorporate and recognise the Treaty, although the initial obligations were revised. This legislation requires District Health Boards to be responsive and address Māori health needs and recognise the Treaty in its decision making and when setting health delivery priorities. This legislation ultimately aims to reduce health disparities and improve Māori health outcomes (Durie, 2011). In addition, the Health Practitioners Competency Assurance Act 2003 requires regulatory authorities to ensure all registered health professionals to demonstrate they are culturally competent when working with people from a different culture than their own.

Māori health workforce development

Article 3 of the Treaty indicates that all Māori should receive the same services as others using the health system, and that every effort should be made to ensure the nature and quality of those services are the same. Being able to connect with the people is vital to improving the health and well-being of whānau and achieving whānau ora. Thus, strengthening the Māori health workforce is imperative as they bring insights and comprehension of the complex cultural and socio-economic issues impacting Māori (Anonson et al., 2008; Hasnain-Wynia et al., 2007; Lloyd et al., 2009).

There is evidence that a health workforce representative of a community's ethnic make up increases the likelihood that indigenous peoples and those belonging to minority groups will use health services (Gilchrist & Rector, 2007). The value of a Māori health workforce can be seen in the role Māori community health workers play – they know their community well, work from a Māori world view and tikanga, and importantly are able to talk the language of the people who live within the community (as opposed to the health jargon used by many health professionals). Despite a concerted effort since 1980 to increase the representation of Māori in the regulated health workforce, little progress has been made to date.

Should a set of cultural competencies for whānau Māori be developed for health practitioners working in New Zealand?

> Should there be implications for non-compliance, similar to clinical competencies?

> Explain the rationale for your responses.

Impact on healthcare practice

Māori experience significant inequities in access to social determinants of health, access to health services and receipt of quality health care. These have all impacted negatively on their health status and health outcomes (Ministry of Health, 2010; Reid & Robson, 2007). Research has shown that Māori are more likely to:

- experience discriminatory behaviours from health practitioners than those identifying as New Zealand European (Harris et al., 2012; Harris et al., 2006a; Harris et al., 2006b; Reid & Robson, 2006);
- experience an adverse event when they do seek hospital care (Davis et al., 2006);
- be hospitalised or die from an amenable or preventable illness (Ministry of Health, 2010).

The Treaty remains central to regulated health profession requirements for cultural safety and cultural competency.

Taking into account the colonial history of New Zealand, should Māori be treated the same as other New Zealanders? If yes, why? If no, why not?

Mulholland and Tawhai (2010) claim the Treaty's relevance has persisted for 173 years. It is a document that will continue to have relevance into the future. Since the 1970s iwi and Māori health professionals and community health workers have asserted their Treaty rights and Māori identity. They have also expressed concerns about the inequities that exist for Māori. Nevertheless, it was not until the mid-1980s, after Māori protests highlighted concerns about the existence of socio-economic, education and health inequalities for Māori compared to others living in New Zealand, that the Treaty featured more prominently on the New Zealand landscape. Over time Māori, using their Treaty rights, have influenced the culture of health services, which has seen the introduction of practices based on tikanga Māori for Māori and their whānau.

The events that led to the signing of the Treaty and the impact that these have had on the health of Māori is evident throughout this chapter.

> What are the continued health risks for whānau Māori?

> What can be done now to mitigate these ongoing negative health outcomes?

Biculturalism

Justice Eddie Durie (2005, p. 1) explains:

> Biculturalism is about the relationship between the state's founding cultures [i.e. Māori and British settlers], where there is more than one.

The concept of biculturalism in Aotearoa New Zealand is premised on the relationship between Māori and the Crown and it establishes Māori rights as the indigenous people of Aotearoa New Zealand. Undoubtedly, New Zealand's population is increasing in its diversity. A common claim made is that the focus should be on multiculturalism not biculturalism. Indeed, a multicultural view facilitates the recognition of diversity among those living in New Zealand. However, the Treaty preserves the bicultural relationship Māori peoples have with Pākehā (European New Zealanders) as the indigenous peoples and as the basis of New Zealand society (Orange, 2004).

Principles of the Treaty

Principles of the Treaty exist to aid interpreting the Treaty's intent (especially because there are two versions of this agreement), the spirit with which it was made and applying these to specific health situations. For example, the Waitangi Tribunal 1975 has a set of principles that it is required to address when it reviews claims (Table 6.2).

The principles of partnership, participation and protection are a set of principles developed by the Royal Commission on Social Policy 1988 and are commonly used within the health setting to underpin health policy, such as

TABLE 6.2 *Waitangi Tribunal Treaty of Waitangi Principles*

PRINCIPLE	MEANING
1. Recognition	Māori and their rangatiratanga
2. Partnership	Equal relationship
3. Options	Choice to live by tikanga Māori and to walk in two worlds
4. Active protection	Crown obligations to reduce disparities
5. Autonomy	Tino rangatiratanga/mana motuhake
6. Rangatiratanga	Right to self-determination

He Korowai Oranga – the Māori Health Strategy (King & Turia, 2002). The development of He Korowai Oranga is an example of the relationship between the Crown and Māori in the health arena that resulted in the collaborative aim of whānau ora . These principles can be used as a framework to guide the way in which health practitioners engage with Māori and their whānau:

- **Partnership** involves establishing meaningful, collaborative relationships with Māori and their whānau. When health practitioners establish relationships with Māori, it can facilitate focusing on hauora (Māori concept of wellness and health), rather than solely on disease or illness. When such partnerships are established, existing strengths that Māori and their whānau possess can be better determined rather than focusing on deficits and negative stereotypes.

- **Participation** consists of including Māori and their whānau in their health care, and all decision making and planning of interventions. Through participation in their health care, Māori have active involvement with health practitioners and their care, rather than being passive recipients of culturally inappropriate or unacceptable care.

- **Protection** is the recognition and respect of Māori the cultural values, beliefs and practices. This involves health practitioners taking steps to include important cultural practices in their health care (for instance, for some Māori it is important for their spiritual well-being that karakia occurs before an intervention). The principle of protection enables cultural affirmation, something that Māori report is missing when they engage with health services (see, for example, Wilson & Barton, 2012), and ignores important cultural beliefs and practices.

These principles can be used as a useful framework to inform health practitioners' practice when they work with Māori and their whānau. It can be also useful for working with people from other cultures. An example of using these three principles in practice is when documenting clinical encounters with Māori and their whānau, and cultural practices negotiated and/or provided in their clinical notes.

Conclusion

Māori are not a homogenous group of people. Diversity exists amongst contemporary Māori, with more Māori claiming ancestry than those who identify ethnically as Māori, and those who have a high level of Māori identity and cultural engagement. Understanding the historical and social impacts on the health of Māori that are associated with the Treaty can facilitate the elimination of biases, assumptions and stereotypes. Equally important is having regard for Māori values and beliefs, and concepts and views of wellness, which can assist in achieving better health outcomes for Māori, although it is important not to assume that all Māori prescribe to the same beliefs.

While health practitioners cannot make an appreciable difference with regard to Māori access to the various social determinants of health, they can influence the access to, and the delivery of, quality health services (Table 6.3). A bicultural practitioner recognises and respects a Māori world view that is holistic, eco-spiritual and relational whereby people have collective orientations and obligations. This differs from the Euro-Western and biomedical views that tend to be reductionist and individually focused. Recognising

TABLE 6.3 *Supporting practice change*

ACTION	EXAMPLES
1. Recognise own biases, assumptions and stereotypes, and how these influence the nature of your practice.	Initiating behaviour change: • organisational culture and environment; • individuals' practices.
2. Understand the historical impacts associated with the Treaty on Māori health today.	Eliminate practice based on stereotypes and unsubstantiated assumptions. Eliminate discriminatory attitudes and behaviours.
3. Engage in meaningful relationships with Māori users of health services and their whānau.	Address power imbalances between Māori users of health services and health practitioners.
4. Recognise Māori ways of wellness.	Become informed. Ask Māori users of health services and their whānau.
5. Facilitate the Treaty right of Māori and their whānau to being actively involved in decision making about their health care.	Involve Māori and their whānau in discussions about their health status, health care and treatment options, and in planning.

one's own biases, assumptions and stereotypes can help to reduce such negative influences when working with whānau Māori and create a safe environment so that open and honest conversations can be had. Nonetheless, strengthening the Māori health workforce is imperative as they bring insights and comprehension of the complex cultural and socio-economic issues impacting Māori.

With regard to the Treaty, is respect for Māori social practices and ways of viewing the world enough to improve the health of whānau Māori?

> If not, what approach would you use and why?

FOR REFLECTION

References

Anonson, J. M., Desjarlais, J., Nixon, J., Whiteman, L. & Bird, A. (2008). Strategies to support recruitment and retention of First Nations youth in baccalaureate nursing programs in Saskatchewan, Canada. *Journal of Transcultural Nursing, 19*(3), 274–83. doi:10.1177/1043659608317095

Confederation of Chiefs of the United Tribes of Aotearoa. (2010). Retrieved 18 November 2014 from http://www.united-tribes.com/history.htm

Davis, P., Lay-Yee, R., Dyall, L., Briant, R., Sporle, A., Brunt, D. & Scott, A. (2006). Quality of hospital care for Māori patients in New Zealand: Retrospective cross-sectional assessment. *The Lancet, 367*(9526), 1920–5. doi:10.1016/s0140–6736(06)68847–8

Dow, D. A. (1999). *Māori health and government policy 1840–1940.* Wellington: Victoria University Press.

Durie, J. (2005). The rule of law, biculturalism and multiculturalism. Paper presented at the meeting of the ALTA Conference, Hamilton. Retrieved 18 November 2014 from http://www.lawcom.govt.nz/sites/default/files/speeches/2005/07/ALTA%20conference%20-%20July%202005%20-%20Durie.pdf

Durie, M. (1998). *Whaiora: Māori health development* (2nd edn.). Auckland: Oxford University Press.

Durie, M. (2001). *Mauri ora: The dynamics of Māori health.* Auckland: Oxford University Press.

Durie, M. (2011). *Ngā tini whetū: Navigating Māori futures.* Wellington: Huia.

Gilchrist, K. L. & Rector, C. (2007). Can you keep them? Strategies to attract and retain nursing students from diverse populations: Best practices in nursing education. *Journal of Transcultural Nursing, 18*(3), 277–85. doi:10.1177/1043659607301305

Harris, R., Cormack, D., Tobias, M., Yeh, L.-C., Talamaivao, N., Minster, J. & Timutimu, R. (2012). The pervasive effects of racism: Experiences of racial discrimination in New Zealand over time and associations with multiple health domains. *Social Science & Medicine, 74*(3), 408–15. doi:10.1016/j. socscimed.2011.11.004

Harris, R., Tobias, M., Jeffreys, M., Waldegrave, K., Karlsen, S. & Nazroo, J. (2006a). Effects of self-reported racial discrimination and deprivation on Māori health and inequalities in New Zealand: Cross-sectional study. *The Lancet, 367*(9527), 2005–9.

Harris, R., Tobias, M., Jeffreys, M., Waldegrave, K., Karlsen, S. & Nazroo, J. (2006b). Racism and health: The relationship between experience of racial discrimination and health in New Zealand. *Social Science & Medicine, 63*(6), 1428–41.

Hasnain-Wynia, R., Baker, D. W., Nerenz, D., Feinglass, J., Beal, A. C., Landrum, M. B., … Weissman, J. S. (2007). Disparities in health care are driven by where minority patients seek care. *JAMA Internal Medicine, 167*(12), 2133–9.

Hunn, J. K. (1960). *Report on Department of Māori Affairs: With statistical supplement.* Wellington: Government Printer.

Ihimaera, W. (ed.). (1998). *Growing up Māori.* Auckland: Tandem Press.

King, A., & Turia, T. (2002). He korowai oranga: Māori health strategy. Wellington: Ministry of Health.

Kingi, T. K. (2005). *The Treaty of Waitangi: 1800–2005.* Paper presented at the meeting of the Te Hui Tauira, Waikawa Marae, Picton. Retrieved 17 November 2014 from http://www.massey.ac.nz/massey/research/centres-research/te-mata-o-te-tau/publications/publications_home.cfm

Kingi, T. K. (2007). The Treaty of Waitangi: A framework for Māori health development. *New Zealand Journal of Occupational Therapy, 54*(1), 4–10.

Lange, R. (1999). *May the people live: A history of Māori health development 1900–1920.* Auckland: Auckland University Press.

Lloyd, J., Wise, M., Weeramanthri, T. & Nugus, P. (2009). The influence of professional values on the implementation of Aboriginal health policy. *Journal of Health Service, Research & Policy, 14*(1), 6–12. doi:10.1258/jhsrp.2008.008002

Ministry of Health. (2010). *Tatau kahukura: Māori health chart book 2010* (2nd edn.). Wellington: Ministry of Health.

Ministry of Health. (2014). *The guide to He Korowai Oranga: Māori Health Strategy 2014.* Wellington: Ministry of Health.

Moon, P. (2003). *Tohunga: Hohepa Kereopa.* Auckland: David Ling Publishing.

Moon, P. (2007). The Treaty of Waitangi: Principles and practice. In D. Broom, B. Deed, K. Dew, M. Durie, J. Germov, A. Kirkman, J. Macdonald, P. Moon, J. Park, B. S. Turner & S. Walke (eds) *Health in the context of Aotearoa New Zealand* (pp. 75–93). Melbourne: Oxford University Press.

Mulholland, M. & Tawhai, V. (2010). *Weeping waters: The Treaty of Waitangi and constitutional change.* Wellington: Huia.

Mutu, M. (2010). Constitutional intentions: The Treaty of Waitangi texts. In M. Mulholland & V. Tawhai (eds) *Weeping waters: The Treaty of Waitangi and constitutional change* (pp. 13–40). Wellington: Huia.

Orange, C. (2004). *An illustrated history of the Treaty of Waitangi*. Wellington: Bridget Williams Books.

Reid, P. & Robson, B. (2006). The state of Māori health. In M. Mulholland (ed.) *State of the Māori nation: Twenty first-century issues in Aotearoa* (pp. 17–32). Auckland: Reed Publishing.

Reid, P. & Robson, B. (2007). Understanding health inequities. In B. Robson & R. Harris (eds) *Hauora: Māori health standards IV. A study of the years 2000–2005* (pp. 3–10). Wellington: Te Ropu Rangahau Hauora a Eru Pomare.

Sinclair, K. (1980). The Māoris in New Zealand history. *History Today series, 30*(7). Retrieved 16 November 2014 from http://www.historytoday.com/keith-sinclair/maoris-new-zealand-history

State Services Commission. (2005). *Timeline of the Treaty*. Wellington: State Services Commission.

Wilson, D. & Barton, P. (2012). Indigenous hospital experiences: A New Zealand case study. *Journal of Clinical Nursing, 21*(15–16), 2316–26. doi:10.1111/j.1365-2702.2011.04042.x

Appendix 1: The Declaration of Independence of New Zealand, 28 October 1835

1. Ko matou, ko nga Tino Rangatira o nga iwi o Nu Tireni i raro mai o Hauraki kua oti nei te huihui i Waitangi i Tokeraui i t era 28 o Oketopa 1835, ka wakaputa i te Rangatiratanga o to matou wenua a ka meatia ka wakaputaia e matou he Wenua Rangatira, kia huaina, Ko te Wakaminenga o nga Hapū o Nu Tireni.

1. We the hereditary chiefs and heads of the tribes of the Northern parts of New Zealand, being assembled at Waitangi, in the Bay of Islands, on this 28th day of October, 1835, declare the Independence of our country, which is hereby constituted and declared to be an Independent State, under the designation of the United Tribes of New Zealand.

2. Ko te Kingitanga ko te mana i te wenua o te wakaminenga o Nu Tireni ka meatia nei kei nga Tino Rangatira anake i to matou huihuinga, a ka mea hoki e kore e tukua e matou te wakarite ture kit e tahi hunga ke atu, me te tahi Kawanatanga hoki kia meatia i te wenua o te wakawakarite ana kit e ritenga o o matou ture e meatia nei matou i to matou huihuinga.

2. All sovereign power and authority within the territories of the united tribes of New Zealand is hereby declared to reside entirely and exclusively in the hereditary chiefs and heads of tribes in their collective capacity, who also declare that they will not permit any legislative authority separate from themselves in their collective capacity to exist, nor any function of government to be exercised within the said territories, unless by persons appointed by them in Congress assembled.

3. Ko matou ko nga tino Rangatira ka mea nei kia huihui kit e runanga ki Waitangi a te Ngahuru I tenei tau I tenei tau kit e wakarite ture kia tika te hokohoko, a ka mea hoki ki nga tauiwi o runga, kia wakarerea te wawai, kia mahara ai ke te wakaoranga o to matou wenua, a kia uru ratou kit e wakaminenga o Nu Tireni.

3. The hereditary chiefs and heads of tribes agree to meet in Congress at Waitangi in the autumn of each year, for the purpose of framing laws for the dispensation of justice, the preservation of peace and good order, and the regulation of trade, and they cordially invite the Southern tribes to lay aside their private animosities and to consult the safety and welfare of our common country, by joining the Confederation of the United Tribes.

4. Ka mea matou kia tuhituhia he pukapuka kite ritenga o tenei o to matou wakaputanga nei ki te Kingi o Ingarani hei kawe atu I to matou aroha nana hoki I wakaae kite kara mo matou. A no te mea aka atawai matou, ka tiaki I nga pākehā e noho nei I uta, e rere mai ana ki te hokohoko, koi aka mea ai matou ki te Kingi kia waiho hei matua I to matou Tamarikitanga kei wakakahoretia to matou Rangatiratanga.

4. They also agree to send a copy of this Declaration to His Majesty, the King of England, to thank him for his acknowledgement of their flag, and in return for his friendship and protection they have shown, and are prepared to show, to such of his subjects as have settled in their country, or resorted to its shores for the purposes of trade, they entreat that he will continue to be the parent of their infant State, and that he will become its protector from all attempts upon its independence.

Kua wakaaetia katoatia e matau I tenei ra I te 28 Oketopa, 1835, ki te aroaro o te Reireneti o te Kingi o Ingarani.

Appendix 2: Te Tiriti o Waitangi – Māori Text

KO WIKITORIA te Kuini o Ingarani i tana mahara atawai ki nga Rangatira me nga Hapū o Nu Tirani i tana hiahia hoki kia tohungia ki a ratou o ratou rangatiratanga me to ratou wenua, a kia mau tonu hoki te Rongo ki a ratou me te Atanoho hoki kua wakaaro ia he mea tika kia tukua mai tetahi Rangatira – hei kai wakarite ki nga Tangata Māori o Nu Tirani – kia wakaaetia e nga Rangatira Māori te Kawanatanga o te Kuini ki nga wahi katoa o te wenua nei me nga motu – na te mea hoki he tokomaha ke nga tangata o tona Iwi kua noho ki tenei wenua, a e haere mai nei.

Na ko te Kuini e hiahia ana kia wakaritea te Kawanatanga kia kaua ai nga kino e puta mai ki te tangata Māori ki te Pākehā e noho ture kore ana.

Na kua pai te Kuini kia tukua a hau a Wiremu Hopihona he Kapitana i te Roiara Nawi hei Kawana mo nga wahi katoa o Nu Tirani e tukua aianei amua atu ki te Kuini, e mea atu ana ia ki nga Rangatira o te wakaminenga o nga hapū o Nu Tirani me era Rangatira atu enei ture ka korerotia nei.

Ko te tuatahi

Ko nga Rangatira o te wakaminenga me nga Rangatira katoa hoki ki hai i uru ki taua wakaminenga ka tuku rawa atu ki te Kuini o Ingarani ake tonu atu – te Kawanatanga katoa o o ratou wenua.

Ko te tuarua

Ko te Kuini o Ingarani ka wakarite ka wakaae ki nga Rangatira ki nga hapū – ki nga tangata katoa o Nu Tirani te tino rangatiratanga o o ratou wenua o ratou kainga me o ratou taonga katoa. Otira ko nga Rangatira o te wakaminenga me nga Rangatira katoa atu ka tuku ki te Kuini te hokonga o era wahi wenua e pai ai te tangata nona te Wenua – ki te ritenga o te utu e wakaritea ai e ratou ko te kai hoko e meatia nei e te Kuini hei kai hoko mona.

Ko te tuatoru

Hei wakaritenga mai hoki tenei mo te wakaaetanga ki te Kawanatanga o te Kuini – Ka tiakina e te Kuini o Ingarani nga tangata Māori katoa o Nu Tirani ka tukua ki a ratou nga tikanga katoa rite tahi ki ana mea ki nga tangata o Ingarani.

(signed) William Hobson, Consul and Lieutenant-Governor.

Na ko matou ko nga Rangatira o te Wakaminenga o nga hapū o Nu Tirani ka huihui nei ki Waitangi ko matou hoki ko nga Rangatira o Nu Tirani ka kite nei i te ritenga o enei kupu, ka tangohia ka wakaaetia katoatia e matou, koia ka tohungia ai o matou ingoa o matou tohu.

Ka meatia tenei ki Waitangi i te ono o nga ra o Pepueri i te tau kotahi mano, e waru rau e wa tekau o to tatou Ariki.

Translation of the Māori Text of Te Tiriti o Waitangi

By Professor Sir Hugh Kawharu (former Treaty of Waitangi Tribunal member) Victoria, the Queen of England, in her concern to protect the chiefs and the subtribes of New Zealand and in her desire to preserve their chieftainship and their lands to them and to maintain peace and good order considers it just to appoint an administrator one who will negotiate with the people of New Zealand to the end that their chiefs will agree to the Queen's Government being established over all parts of this land and (adjoining) islands and also because there are many of her subjects already living on this land and others yet to come. So the Queen desires to establish a government so that no evil will come to Māori and European living in a state of lawlessness. So the Queen has appointed 'me, William Hobson a Captain' in the Royal Navy to be Governor for all parts of New Zealand (both those) shortly to be received by the Queen and (those) to be received hereafter and presents to the chiefs of the Confederation chiefs of the subtribes of New Zealand and other chiefs these laws set out here.

The first

The Chiefs of the Confederation and all the Chiefs who have not joined that Confederation give absolutely to the Queen of England for ever the complete government over their land.

The second

The Queen of England agrees to protect the chiefs, the subtribes and all the people of New Zealand in the unqualified exercise of their chieftainship over their lands, villages and all their treasures. But on the other hand the Chiefs of the Confederation and all the Chiefs will sell land to the Queen at a price agreed to by the person owning it and by the person buying it (the latter being) appointed by the Queen as her purchase agent.

The third

For this agreed arrangement therefore concerning the Government of the Queen, the Queen of England will protect all the ordinary people of New Zealand and will give them the same rights and duties of citizenship as the people of England.

[signed] William Hobson Consul & Lieut Governor

So we, the Chiefs of the Confederation of the subtribes of New Zealand meeting here at Waitangi having seen the shape of these words which we accept and agree to record our names and our marks thus.

Was done at Waitangi on the sixth of February in the year of our Lord 1840.

Appendix 3: The Treaty of Waitangi – English text

HER MAJESTY VICTORIA Queen of the United Kingdom of Great Britain and Ireland regarding with Her Royal Favour the Native Chiefs and Tribes of New Zealand and anxious to protect their just Rights and Property and to secure to them the enjoyment of Peace and Good Order has deemed it necessary in consequence of the great number of Her Majesty's Subjects who have already settled in New Zealand and the rapid extension of Emigration both from Europe and Australia which is still in progress to constitute and appoint a functionary properly authorised to treat with the Aborigines of New Zealand for the recognition of Her Majesty's Sovereign authority over the whole or any part of those islands – Her Majesty therefore being desirous to establish a settled form of Civil Government with a view to avert the evil consequences which must result from the absence of the necessary Laws and Institutions alike to the native population and to Her subjects has been graciously pleased to empower and to authorise me William Hobson a Captain in Her Majesty's Royal Navy Consul and Lieutenant-Governor of such parts of New Zealand as may be or hereafter shall be ceded to her Majesty to invite the confederated and independent Chiefs of New Zealand to concur in the following Articles and Conditions.

Article the first [Article 1]

The Chiefs of the Confederation of the United Tribes of New Zealand and the separate and independent Chiefs who have not become members of the Confederation cede to Her Majesty the Queen of England absolutely and without reservation all the rights and powers of Sovereignty which the said Confederation or Individual Chiefs respectively exercise or possess, or may be supposed to exercise or to possess over their respective Territories as the sole sovereigns thereof.

Article the second [Article 2]

Her Majesty the Queen of England confirms and guarantees to the Chiefs and Tribes of New Zealand and to the respective families and individuals thereof the full exclusive and undisturbed possession of their Lands and Estates Forests Fisheries and other properties which they may collectively or individually possess so long as it is their wish and desire to retain the same in their possession; but the Chiefs of the United Tribes and the individual Chiefs yield to Her Majesty the exclusive right of Pre-emption over such lands as the proprietors thereof may be disposed to alienate at such prices as may be agreed upon between the respective Proprietors and persons appointed by Her Majesty to treat with them in that behalf.

Article the third [Article 3]

In consideration thereof Her Majesty the Queen of England extends to the Natives of New Zealand Her royal protection and imparts to them all the Rights and Privileges of British Subjects.

(signed) William Hobson, Lieutenant-Governor.

Now therefore We the Chiefs of the Confederation of the United Tribes of New Zealand being assembled in Congress at Victoria in Waitangi and We the Separate and Independent Chiefs of New Zealand claiming authority over the Tribes and Territories which are specified after our respective names, having been made fully to understand the Provisions of the foregoing Treaty, accept and enter into the same in the full spirit and meaning thereof in witness of which we have attached our signatures or marks at the places and the dates respectively specified. Done at Waitangi this Sixth day of February in the year of Our Lord one thousand eight hundred and forty.

7

Exploring prejudice, understanding paradox and working towards new possibilities

Deb Spence

Learning objectives

Having studied this chapter, you will be able to:

- recognise how the past influences the present and the future (both personal and professional);

- consider prejudices (pre-understandings) as enabling and limiting;

- understand the contradictory nature of healthcare delivery;

- question current practice in order to see new and different future possibilities.

Key terms and concepts

- cultural difference

- cultural identity

- new possibilities

- paradox (in nursing)

- prejudice

- tension (in nursing)

Introduction

> It is not enough to understand what we ought to be unless we know what we are;
> And we do not understand what we are, unless we know what we ought to
> be. (T. S. Eliot, 1935)

T. S. Eliot reminds us of the relationship between our beliefs and values, and our interactions, interpretations and responses. He also describes the inextricable interrelationship of past, present, and future events and meanings. Exploring past and present meanings of 'culture' in the context of New Zealand nursing is an essential part of future development. This chapter begins by tracing the evolving meaning of culture within the context of New Zealand nursing. It then describes the meaning of cultural difference from a nursing perspective and explores the notions of prejudice, paradox and possibility in relation to nursing practice.

Nurses in New Zealand have experienced considerable public criticism for their efforts towards a fairer and more equitable health service. The introduction of cultural safety in nursing and midwifery education has been, and continues to be, the subject of much debate. Nursing people from cultures other than one's own is a complex and contradictory undertaking and 'striving towards right', in this context, lives in the tensions and prejudices of nursing practice. Success is achieved when possibilities are recognised and the nurse and the person from another culture understand each other.

Evolutions in meaning

The literature provides evidence that the meaning of the term 'culture' in nursing has changed significantly in recent decades (Morse, 1988; Spence, 2001a). Early associations with 'racial' physicality were replaced initially by anthropological understandings and subsequently moved to encompass a more socio-political awareness of the consequences of a monocultural health service for those of indigenous and/or minority status. The growing significance of biculturalism has been an important catalyst but New Zealand nurses, like their international colleagues, also understand cultural differences to be broader than ethnic difference. Against a dynamic and evolving background of meanings, they are extending their understandings of culture.

Cultural difference in nursing

Nurses understand people from other cultures in relation to themselves, that is, as different from 'me', in both a personal sense and in terms of group membership. A name, the language spoken, skin colour, dress and gestures are noticed and not taken for granted in the way that they might be in encounters with people from one's own culture. Encountering difference means experiencing one's self as a nurse in relation to a person who is 'culturally other'. It means noticing the patient as different, yet similar to other patients in terms of their need for nursing. Paradoxically then, it means simultaneously engaging with similarity and difference.

Interpreting difference to mean Māori

Drawing from the findings of doctoral research that explored the experience of nursing people from other cultures in New Zealand, Amanda, a research participant, speaks of being:

> ... more acutely aware for Māori people ... I'm trying to make an effort ... Yes. I really want to be part of this country so I believe I have to put in effort ... I feel accountable because if we have a Treaty and are saying this, then I feel I have to uphold my end of it. (Research participant, in Spence, 1999, p. 143)

Amanda was born in New Zealand and describes herself as a Pākehā New Zealander. Underpinning her nursing efforts is an awareness of bicultural issues and responsibility in terms of the Treaty of Waitangi. Despite the burgeoning ethnic diversity of New Zealand's population, there is heightened awareness of the need to redress the differences experienced by Māori in terms of health inequalities.

Other differences that matter

In addition to ethnicity, difference has meaning in relation to gender, age, social class and occupation. Cultural variations relating to rural and urban socialisation experiences are also recognised.

> This is generalising a bit, but people who live in Auckland seem to be more forward about asking or telling you that something's not right ... people from the little towns ... just sit there quietly ...

> Epsom has a culture of its own. They expect you there at 9am and if you're not there by five past, they're on the phone finding out where you are. (Research participant, in Spence, 1999, p. 101)

Questioning the relationship between identity and difference

What then is the meaning of cultural difference? Can a person's uniqueness be identified separately from who they are culturally and historically as a group? If individuals are all so different, what is cultural identity?

Having attempted to explore what she means by culture in her journal, Anne, another research participant (Spence, 1999, p. 106), writes: 'Mores, attitudes, beliefs, habits, world-view, spiritual beliefs, attitudes towards women and men, children, childbirth?'

However, there is more from a nursing perspective, so she decides:

> I would put well-being above everything, like self-esteem, not disempowering a person. Cultural identity is part of that. Sometimes it's very hard to know what cultural identity is. How do I know what a Somali's cultural identity is? I might read a lot about them and that may help but when it comes to communication between you and the person, you can have all the knowledge in the world and be absolutely hopeless.

Cultural identity is being tentatively defined to include the beliefs and practices generally adopted by those from the same country. Yet Anne knows that she is unlikely to ever possess the relevant cultural knowledge and she believes that nursing relationships need to be based on more than cross-cultural understanding of this type. Although she recognises that knowledge of others' cultural practices is helpful, she also knows that such knowledge is useless in the hands of nurses who are not respectful of patients as individual persons. The other person's cultural identity is important because of its contribution to self-esteem. Anne tries, therefore, to ensure that her actions do not disempower the other person. Of greatest importance is an attitude that acknowledges and respects difference.

> I try to get through to the essence of the person, transcending cultural barriers. Most of it is an overall sensitivity that tries to foster respect and openness. Only part is cultural. (Research participant, in Spence, 1999, p. 106)

The inextricable relationship between individual and cultural identity is a constant source of tension in nursing because nurses are continually confronted with culture both in an individual sense and in terms of group meaning. On balance, their conclusion is that individual identity is greater than, but inclusive of, one's socially prescribed cultural identity.

> I don't think you can separate them. A person's culture is part of who they are. You have to deal with all aspects together . . .

> Culture is your very being . . . It's not just what a person is at that time. It's their past and their future and what they are. (Research participants, in Spence, 1999, p. 107)

Difference as difficulty

Nurses experience greater uncertainty when nursing people from other cultures. Difference has meaning in terms of difficulty in nursing because the nurse cannot assume that the patient will share, or be able to understand, the values and beliefs that inform nursing practice. In addition to experiencing 'difference from me' in a personal sense and as a member of a cultural group, cultural difference is problematic because of its potential to restrict communication and its challenge to institutional mores. People from other cultures are also often perceived to be more vulnerable by nurses. Thus a greater need to communicate and establish trust exists alongside the increased difficulty of achieving this.

A mental health experience

Practice example 1

I must admit my first encounter with a Polynesian patient was quite hair raising. I had to go and do a blood pressure on a very psychotic and paranoid young man. He was big – about 20 stone. He was a gang member with patches on. And he had dreadlocks. I mean dreadlocks to me is Rastafarian and in England that sort of population brought fear to me. It was a nightmare. I had never encountered anything like this before. My hands were clammy. I had to keep telling myself 'Look this is within your professional capacity. You'll be all right. If anything happens there'll be other staff who will come to your rescue.' I kept telling myself, 'It'll be fine. It'll be fine. Just remember your psychiatric skills. Talk to the person.' In my mind's eye I recalled telling my son that when he came into contact with a growling dog, 'Don't show you're afraid', and I kind of related to that. 'Don't show your fear. Just get on with it.' But I didn't feel safe. I wanted to be a million miles away. It was very hard.

I suppose the charge nurse thought I'd get on better with him because I had a brown face and maybe for him my brown face was OK. But the moment I opened my mouth, with this really prominent English accent, the poor man was quite confused. 'There's somebody speaking. It's not your voice.' And a job that should have taken five minutes took more than half an hour.

I explained the procedure, sort of jabbering along to cover up my fear and hoping he wouldn't pick up that my hands were trembling. It took a lot of encouragement and persuasion. Then later, after we had built up a rapport, he told me how confusing it had been for him and when he improved he came up to me and said, 'Hey Sue. You're a bit staunch, but you're all right'.

This vignette is reproduced from Spence, D. G. (2001). Hermeneutic notions illuminate cross-cultural nursing experiences. Journal of Advanced Nursing, 35, *624–30 with permission © 2001 John Wiley & Sons Ltd.*

FOR REFLECTION

› How are past understandings influencing decision making in this scenario?
› What enables the nurse to establish a relationship with this person?

Prejudices as enabling and limiting

Nurses, like all human beings, come to embody the values and expectations of those with whom they interact through processes of socialisation. Gadamer (1996) uses the term 'prejudice' to describe the unconscious judgements or pre-understandings that influence all interpretation. In defining prejudice as a 'judgement that is rendered before all the elements that determine a situation have been fully examined', Gadamer (1996, p. 270) challenges the negativity associated with its contemporary usage and suggests that adequate understanding needs to include both positive and negative meanings. More important, however, is the recognition that some prejudices are 'true' in the sense that they make ongoing development of understanding possible while others are 'false' because they constrain/ or preclude the development of new and different understandings. Appropriating Gadamer's interpretation to the nursing context, I believe there is much to be gained by understanding the origins of certain prejudices. It is also important to identify those that enable and those that constrain so that questions can be asked about the value or otherwise of continuing practices that may no longer be appropriate.

Enabling prejudices allows:

- a willingness to provide assistance to those in need;
- belief in equal rights to equal standards of care;
- engaging with difference in order to extend one's understanding;
- questioning one's own beliefs and expectations;
- seeking permission;
- being able to listen without interrupting;
- imaginatively placing oneself in the position of another;
- practising holistically;
- 'being with' and 'being present';
- advocating for patients when required.

Limiting prejudices causes:

- fear or avoidance of contact with difference;
- belief in the superiority of Western medicine;
- assumed understanding without checking its accuracy;
- being too busy to listen;
- focusing on 'self' rather than 'other';

- expectations of others to comply with your beliefs and values;
- doing what is minimally necessary;
- prioritising technical skill over interpersonal skill.

Understanding paradox in health care

Paradox refers to the coexistence of apparent opposites and, more specifically, describes situations which, initially seeming to be incongruent, prove on closer examination to have foundation.

When nursing people from cultures other than one's own, paradox describes the dynamic interplay of numerous tensions. For example, nurses expect and are expected by others to reach out to and provide specialised assistance to people needing their skills. Patients (or clients) bring particular values and expectations to the nursing encounter and likewise interpret their experiences against a background of meaning. Thus each and every individual encounter is uniquely different. Each person derives different understandings from their situation and yet, paradoxically, interdependent and common understandings are also possible. Similarity coexists with difference.

Arguing that nursing practice must be 'culturally safe', as defined by the client, Ramsden (1997) challenges the International Council of Nurses' Code of Ethics for seeming to deny difference, suggesting that people should be nursed 'regardful of all that makes them unique, rather than regardless of colour or creed'. The challenge is indeed valid. But are these philosophies necessarily anti-ethical?

The following couplet by Pat Parker (1978, p. 68) exemplifies the paradoxical nature of respect for difference:

> The first thing you do is forget that I'm black,
> Second, you must never forget that I'm black.

Winnicott (1974, p. xiii) asks for 'paradox to be accepted, tolerated and respected for it is not to be resolved' yet such acceptance does not imply passivity. I believe that it is only through consciously and carefully exploring contradictory positions that understanding deepens. Efforts to reduce or suppress conflict risk failing to recognise the necessity of conflict for growth (Miller, 1985).

Alice's story

Practice example 2

I particularly remember looking after a Lebanese gentleman and his family. He had come in with an acute illness and a potentially fatal prognosis and neither he nor his wife spoke a lot of English, although they understood a limited amount. Their sons spoke and understood English well.

I noticed that any staff involved in looking after this man seemed to get pulled into a very intense caring relationship with the family – more intense than I've seen with other cultures – and I didn't think it was just them as individuals. It seemed to me that people from that part of Europe or the Middle East were more passionate – their facial expressions – they wanted so much. They were what I call 'emotional people', wearing their hearts on their sleeves, and I wondered if looking after Italian people might be similar.

What really struck me was that there were no resources. I didn't know who or where to turn to for information on how to care for these people in a cultural sense. They seemed easily offended. If you didn't accept food when they offered it to you, no matter how fast you were speeding down the ward, or how many drips or things you had in your hands, they got very offended. It was almost as if they wanted you to really like them because if you didn't, they thought they wouldn't get good care. And maybe where they come from, that is what happens.

Then, for a time, I couldn't look after this man. He had developed some nasty infections that placed my other patients at risk. But trying to explain this to the family – that it wasn't that I didn't want to look after him – they were very hurt and wouldn't talk to me. I'm sure there was a major cultural component. It was more than a family in grief. I knew they didn't understand and I tried to support them. But time, in work hours, didn't allow searching for things and it wasn't the interpreter service that I needed. I felt I needed to be better prepared.

In this story, difference has meaning in terms of the greater demands perceived to be being made on the nursing staff by this family. Alice experiences tension in the form of feelings of confusion, frustration and guilt. Aware that she does not understand the meaning of the family's expressions, she wants to find resources to assist. Like the family, she too strives to be understood and liked, yet she is unable to help and feels harshly judged because the family cannot understand her position.

The prejudices constraining cross-cultural understanding outweigh those that enable. Alice seems to assume that, because the sons are fluent in English, the family should be able to understand and accept the priorities and practices of the healthcare system with which they are engaging. Although there is evidence that Alice questions her interpretation of the family's more passionate expressions, she attributes greater significance to cultural difference than to the possibly universal emotional pain of a potentially fatal prognosis. Thus, in interpreting their behaviour in terms of difference, she paradoxically sees, but does not see, the family's pain. Furthermore, in seeking resources to improve her knowledge of cultural difference, Alice seems to have overlooked the potential for her relationship with the family to provide this information. Her busyness with 'drips and things' and fears of 'infection risk' appear to have unwittingly precluded the development of trust with this family. Perhaps, in prioritising medical science and technology, Alice is underplaying the importance of human care processes in nursing (Watson, 1988).

Forrest (1989) notes that when situations become difficult, nurses often distance themselves from the patient by providing limited or routine physical care. In 'being busy' one can avoid the deeper and more challenging levels of involvement. Yet it is only when we strive to understand others' perspectives that we can begin to discover concerns that are critically important to us as well (Taylor, 1994).

Working towards new possibilities for practice

Possibility acknowledges the infinite nature of human understanding (Spence, 2001b). It describes potentialities that are diverse where there is openness to new or different understandings and practice. Gadamer (1996) suggests that the person who is ready and able to listen is fundamentally open. Such readiness opens the possibility for entering the 'play', a questioning and enquiring which is directed towards escaping from constraining prejudices. Possibility recognises that tensions, misunderstandings and distortions are always inherent in interpretation but this does not mean that new and different understandings cannot be achieved. Nor does the infinite nature of the process mean that such engagement is without value because movement between opposites is an inevitable part of being human (Reason & Rowan, 1981).

When nursing people from other cultures, possibility means being alive to the way understanding shapes, disrupts and facilitates practice. It means being willing to wonder, being open to positive and negative judgements, and being able to scrutinise and change practice. The possibility of coming to understand others and of continuing one's self-development arises through willing engagement with people who are culturally different. Striving towards right (Spence, 2004) requires responding consciously and unconsciously on multiple levels. It means striving towards others because one is called upon to do so. It also means striving to implement and maintain professional ideals and seeking, where possible, to extend these to the wider community.

Encouraging cross-cultural understanding

Practice example 3

A Pākehā family asked, 'How long are those people going to be next door? It stinks.' So I talked about it with them saying: 'Well that's what they want to do and you're doing what you want to do.' And they were quite surprised and said: 'We're not doing anything to offend them.' And I said, 'How do you know that?' And they said, 'Why should we be?' – so I explained.

'You might like to know that they're staying in their room because they're too embarrassed to come into the lounge.'

'Why would they be embarrassed?'

'Because they see that you are there.'

So in the end they said, 'Well we don't want that', and I went to their room and said, 'The people next door would be happy if you want to come into the lounge but she's feeling a bit sick because of the smell of your Kentucky Fried Chicken.'

So they said, 'Oh, OK. We'll eat it up and then come through.'

And everyone sat there quite happily. Afterwards the Pākehā husband said to me, 'They were really quite nice weren't they?'

> ❭ What are the tensions inherent in this scenario?
> ❭ How does the nurse facilitate a resolution?

FOR REFLECTION

Conclusion

In this chapter I have argued the importance of identifying, exploring and questioning the paradoxes encountered in practice. The old adage that human beings have two ears and one mouth and that one should therefore listen twice as often as one speaks is sage advice. Statements such as: 'I'm convinced you've never got it sussed' (Spence, 1999, p. 177) encapsulate the contradictory nature of healthcare practice; however, being willing to listen and learn, trying to be flexible and gently but rigorously questioning personal and institutional assumptions, help to achieve positive outcomes. As is reiterated by Gadamer (1996), the art is seeing what is questionable, and to this I would add that there is an art to questioning in ways that make new understandings possible.

Acknowledgements removed for this revision.

References

Eliot, T. S. (1935). Religion and literature. In R. T. T. Tripp, (1981) (ed.) *The International Thesaurus of Quotations*. Harmondsworth: Penguin.

Forrest, D. (1989). The experience of caring. *Journal of Advanced Nursing, 14*, 815–23.

Gadamer, H. G. (1996). *Truth and method* (2nd rev. edn.), translated by J. Weinsheimer & D. Marshall. New York: Continuum.

Miller, J. B. (1985). *The necessity of conflict*. New York: Harrington Park Press.

Morse, J. M. (1988). *Recent advances in nursing: Cross-cultural nursing*. Edinburgh: Churchill Livingstone.

Parker, P. (1978). For the white person who wants to be my friend. In *Movements in black: Collected poetry of Pat Parker*. New York: Firebrand Books.

Ramsden, I. (1997). Cultural safety: Implementing the concept. The social force of nursing and midwifery. In P. Te Whaiti, M. McCarthy & A. Durie (eds) *Maii Rangiatea*. Auckland: Auckland University Press, Bridget Williams Books.

Reason, P. & Rowan, J. (1981). *Human Inquiry*. New York: John Wiley and Sons.

Spence, D. G. (1999). Prejudice, paradox and possibility: Nursing people from cultures other than one's own. Unpublished PhD thesis, Massey University, Palmerston North.

Spence, D. G. (2001a). The evolving meaning of 'culture' in New Zealand nursing. *Nursing Praxis in New Zealand, 17*(3), 51–61.

Spence, D. G. (2001b). Prejudice, paradox and possibility: Nursing people from cultures other than one's own. *Journal of Transcultural Nursing, 12*(2), 100–6.

Spence, D. G. (2004). Prejudice, paradox and possibility: The experience of nursing people from cultures other than one's own. In K. H. Kavanagh & V. Knowlden (eds) *Many voices: Towards caring culture in healthcare and healing*. Wisconsin: University of Wisconsin Press.

Taylor, C. (1994). Philosophical reflections on caring practices. In S. Phillips & P. Benner (eds) *The crisis of care: Affirming and restoring caring practices in the helping professions*. Washington: University Press.

Watson, J. (1988). *Nursing: Human science and human care*. New York: National League for Nursing.

Winnicott, D. W. (1974). *Playing and reality*. Harmondsworth: Penguin.

8 Navigating the ethics in cultural safety

Ruth De Souza

Learning objectives

Having studied this chapter, you will be able to:

- explore how ethics requires health professionals to consider and reconsider those 'taken for granted';

- examine how you can respond ethically to clients whose culture might be different from your own;

- consider how your own cultural history and experiences impact on the client's cultural practices;

- consider the assumptions and values of the biomedical model of health;

- review dominant ethical frameworks used in health;

- consider alternative ethical models.

Key terms and concepts

- autonomy
- cultural safety
- decision making
- ethic of care
- ethics
- harm
- justice
- moral imperialism
- relativism
- universalism
- virtue ethics

Introduction

Caring is an ethical activity with a deep moral commitment that relies on a trusting relationship (Holstein, 2001). Health professionals are expected to be caring, skilful, and knowledgeable providers of appropriate and effective care to vulnerable people. Through universal services they are expected to meet the needs of both individual clients and broader communities, which are activities requiring sensitivity and responsiveness. In an increasingly complex globalised world, ethical reflection is required so that practitioners can recognise plurality: in illness explanations; in treatment systems; in the varying roles of family/whānau or community in decision making; and in the range of values around interventions and outcomes. To work effectively in multiple contexts, practitioners must be able to morally locate their practice in both historical legacies of their institutional world and the diversifying community environment. This chapter examines the frameworks that health professionals can use for cross-cultural interactions. I then explore how they can select the most appropriate one depending on the person or group being cared for.

Ethics

Ethics is a part of all our actions as humans and as nurses. Ethics is about how nurses talk to their clients, how they respond to difference and how they make decisions. The word originates from the Greek word 'ethos', which refers to habits and character. Ethics can be seen in all religions, philosophies and cultures, even in those language groups that do not use the term. In the context of health, having an ethical framework provides a shared means of collectively and systematically examining varying viewpoints related to moral questions of right and wrong. Ethics is also a generic term used to refer to the ways people can think about, understand and examine how best to live a 'moral life' (Beauchamp & Childress, 2001). Ethics involves critical thinking and asking questions to highlight the appropriate course of action. It requires health professionals to consider and reconsider the taken for granted (Beauchamp & Childress, 1983). When working with people, it is inevitable that health professionals will confront an 'ethical problem' – a situation that raises questions that cannot be answered with a simple rule or fact. How do health professionals know what they 'ought' to do in a situation? On what ethical grounds or with what criteria do they make their decisions?

Culture, ethics and health

Culture guides our moral decisions in life and morals are expressed differently within and between cultures. Health professionals are required to respond ethically to the needs of clients whose culture might be distinct from their own. Just as a pharmaceutical prescription will vary among clients, whose existing conditions would yield varying effects for the same dose, so too will the same action of care yield different effects for different clients. This is true for all clients, not only the visibly different. Clients are separated from their cultural resources and contexts when they enter a health service. When treated in a Western medical healthcare system, they become members of a distinct patient subculture (Yarbrough & Klotz, 2007, p. 500) and cannot provide for themselves within an institutional environment (Woods, 2010, p. 719). Thus health professionals are confronted with the tension of attempting to provide culturally responsive care to clients with whom they may not share the same values or beliefs. Cultural diversity and globalisation only intensify the ancient tension between moral universalism and moral cultural relativism (Melé & Sánchez-Runde, 2013, p. 681).

Ethics provide a way of negotiating different perspectives in health. They involve a systematic approach to understanding, analysing and distinguishing matters of right and wrong, and following a course of action as a result. In the field of biomedical ethics, seemingly neutral and universal principles are used to navigate through ethical dilemmas to reach value-free answers (Doane 2002, p. 521). Using such principles allows health professionals to go beyond their own beliefs and values to consider the needs of others. Yet, at the interface of care, complex relations of social and cultural power make biomedical neutrality impossible. Professionals instead have to work to recognise power relations that structure the healthcare encounter, relations that may be instituted by social and cultural forces that exceed any individual. Consequently, empowering practices rely on a social justice framework in order for power imbalances to be addressed. The ability to consider the social and cultural needs of the recipient of care, rather than blindly reproducing that of the healthcare system, is at the heart of the ethical encounter. To effectively respond to the gap in those needs requires professionals to understand the cultural assumptions of their own context.

Ethics must consider how general philosophical principles reflect the needs of members from particular communities. In particular, it must look at how cultural and religious traditions play a part in shaping experiences of birth, illness, ageing and death (Turner 2003, p. 102) and consider cross-cultural variations in what constitutes ethical healthcare practice. What is considered responsible and caring in one culture might be viewed as uncaring and callous in another (2003, p. 102).

Cross-cultural differences

One Saturday, when I was working a daytime shift on a postnatal ward, a fellow midwife used a client's young son to interpret for his mother because 'interpreters cost a lot of money at the weekend'. I was shocked and upset when I heard the midwife ask the boy to ask his mother how much blood was on her maternity pad.

FOR REFLECTION

This practice example shows how an issue that can be resolved practically, can have profound ethical, familial and social implications.

› Is it appropriate for a gendered, generational, social and intimate boundary to be crossed for convenience and economy?

› What circumstances would make it acceptable?

Assumptions of the biomedical health model

As stated earlier in the chapter, one of the ways that professionals can increase their capacity to be culturally 'safe' is to ensure that they consider the ways in which their values impact on care. This section, therefore, considers some of the values and assumptions of the dominating force of biomedicine in Western health care. In a thoughtful critique of biomedicine (Ornelas 2008, p. 186), the central assumptions of biomedicine are:

- the weight of authority carried by biomedical technologies over more inter-personal interventions;
- the emphasis on crisis and cure over prevention;
- the dominance of physical interventions to rid the body of observable illness and disease.

Ornelas notes that the dominance of biomedical healing technologies reflects cultural norms of the dominant culture that infuse policies and procedures. The Hippocratic tradition emerged from relatively homogenous societies that gave rise to the European Romantic culture of individualism. Biomedicine reflects this history by exerting an individualising force on practitioners and clients at the expense of communal interventions. Yet biomedicine is only one of many world views that explain suffering. Symptoms, illnesses and interventions do not have the same meaning or impact for people from different cultural backgrounds. Beliefs and values about illness causation can include that illness is a result of the transgression of morality, the interpersonal, the psychological, the socio-political or intrapsychic.

Ornelas concludes that the dominance of biomedicine, at the expense of other views of illness causation, means that care can be unequally distributed and biased in medical decision making. Dominant diagnostic categories, procedures and interventions have been developed and defined in terms of the cultural norms, values, and assumptions of dominant groups. This has enabled the relevance of the client's cultural background to be maximised (stereotyped) or minimised (ignored). For this reason, it is important to understand the historical development of dominant ethical frameworks.

Dominant ethical frameworks

Deontology emerged from the Greek term *deon* for 'binding duty'. It is a theory of doing the right thing and giving equal respect to everyone. This theory is derived from Western religious ethics and based on duties, rights and rules: the focus is on acts rather than the consequences of those acts. An example of this theory is Kant's 'categorical imperative' – the idea that you should only do unto others as you would have them do to you. A fundamental assumption of this theory is that people are autonomous and their personhood is as valuable as the next person, and therefore their humanity should be respected in an absolute fashion. It can be seen at the basis of human rights. For example, the *Universal Declaration of Human Rights* (United Nations, 1948) claims: 'All human beings are born free and equal in dignity and rights.' One problem with this notion is that it raises questions such as: if everyone has the right to the highest attainable standard of health, are they equally entitled to it regardless of cost or benefit to broader society?

Another example of deontological ethics can be found in codes of practice. Professional values contained in the code of ethics guide professionals in how they ought to be and behave. This is known as 'ethical objectivism'. The Code of Conduct for Nurses ('the Code of Conduct'), for example, is a set of standards by the Nursing Council of New Zealand ('the Nursing Council') (2012) providing guidance on appropriate behaviour for all nurses.

Reflecting on the scenario that opened this chapter, as someone new to working in maternity and feeling like I had very little power, the incident I described confronted me with an everyday ethical dilemma. At the time I believed that it was inappropriate for a child (let alone a male child) to interpret for his mother, particularly because of the personal nature of the information that was being requested. At the time I had far fewer skills than I have now for intervening in the situation or for advocating for the mother and her child. However, while my experience of the ethical situation was personal, there are resources in codes of conduct that could assist me in resolving the dilemma.

The Code of Conduct requires that nurses:

- 1.2 Take steps to ensure the physical environment allows health consumers to maintain their privacy and dignity.
- 2.7 Assist the health consumer to gain appropriate support and representation from those who understand the health consumer's first-language, culture, needs and preferences.
- 3.4 Meet health consumers' language and communication needs where reasonably practicable.
- 6.9 Intervene to stop unsafe, incompetent, unethical or unlawful practice. Discuss the issues with those involved. Report to an appropriate person at the earliest opportunity and take other actions necessary to safeguard health consumers.
- 6.10 Use a recognised ethical code or framework to assist you and your colleagues in ethical decision making, for example, New Zealand Nurses Organisation (2013) *Code of Ethics*.
- 7.2 Protect vulnerable health consumers from exploitation and harm.
- 7.3 Act promptly if a health consumer's safety is compromised (Nursing Council of New Zealand, 2012, pp. 7–33).

The *Code of Health and Disability Services Consumers' Rights* (Health and Disability Commissioner, 1996) grants a number of rights to all consumers of health and disability services in New Zealand, and places obligations to service providers.

Right 1: the right to be treated with respect.

Right 3: the right to dignity and independence.

Right 4: the right to services of an appropriate standard.

Right 8: the right to support.

Right 10: the right to complain.

A criticism of codes of ethics is that they can be broad and non-specific meaning that everyday ethical challenges are inadequately addressed. On the other hand their value lies in the recognition of diverse contexts, where moral rules cannot be specified in advance, and nurses in those contexts need freedom to develop their moral judgement. Therefore, the existence of such codes is not a guarantee of ethical behaviour but a resource that practitioners can use to support their ethical enquiry.

Consequentialism

A second dominant tradition in Western philosophical ethics is consequentialism. A theory holds that people should do whatever leads to the best consequences for the greatest number of people by focusing on real consequences instead of intentions, or ends, rather than means. The principle of utility means that the morally right thing in any situation is to do the action that promotes the maximisation of happiness and minimisation of suffering for most people. It avoids some of the challenges that come with deontological approaches, such as respecting the freedom to those who will undertake destructive acts. However, one of the critiques of utilitarian or consequentialist approaches is that terrible things can be justified because one is more focused on the end result, yet when this 'end' is and who will judge it remains uncertain.

Principlism

Principlism is a dominant framework for ethical decision making and problem solving in Western bioethics that ranges across deontological and consequentialist approaches. Principlism forms the basis for the *Code of Ethics* developed by the New Zealand Nurses Organisation (2013).

In the Anglo-American tradition it has been developed by Beauchamp and Childress (1983). This framework utilises four purportedly universal principles:

autonomy, beneficence, nonmaleficence and justice; with individual autonomy viewed as foundational (Johnstone & Kanitsaki, 2009, p. 408). A European version of principilism, exemplified in the Barcelona Declaration (1998), adopts autonomy, dignity, integrity and vulnerability as its basic principles, considering autonomy in a less individualistic and more socially integrated fashion. The idea in both cases is that these principles can be universally considered in ways that more rule-bound versions of deontological ethics cannot.

However, critics like Delany and colleagues (2013) question whether Western developed bioethical frameworks can provide universal approaches to ethics or whether they constitute moral imperialism[1], given that they largely ignore multiple cultural and religious traditions. The principles of beneficence, avoidance of harm, autonomy and justice can frequently be thought to only apply to a single person (Delany et al., 2013, p. 72). Cultural critiques of individual autonomy subjugate it to family decision making and collective values including harmony and interdependence (Delany et al., 2013, p. 13; Johnstone & Kanitsaki, 2009, p. 410). Autonomy can be isolating and, for those who are already carrying the burden of illness, a barrier to making choices. Hence, decisions made collaboratively by a family, for instance, would be more valued than individual decision making. However this requires health professionals to understand the importance of family self-determination and to take into account a patient's culture. Thus the patient may be making an autonomous choice by choosing to delegate authority to family, who then takes responsibility or carries the burden of advocacy and protection. The *Code of Ethics* acknowledges the need for nurses to appreciate that autonomy can be both individual and collective (whānau, hapū, iwi).

There are alternative ethical models which are less concerned with conforming to normative principles, ethical duties and rules, or predictable consequences of particular actions for practice. These include virtue ethics, an ethic of care and cultural safety.

Virtue ethics

Virtue ethics focuses on theories that emphasise the role of moral character or virtue of the person carrying out an action rather than the action itself. Based on Aristotle's writings (384–382 BCE), virtue ethics is concerned with moral character, or habits of excellence, or skilled disposition that enable a person to

---

[1] Moral imperialism is the imposition of a set of moral values onto a culture that does not share those values, either through force or through cultural criticism (Jenkins, 2011, p.721).

be good, live a good life and flourish. If you have a 'good' character you will behave ethically. Attaining happiness (eudaimonia) is achieved by performing rational activities (thinking) and through excellence in choosing the mean between extremes, that is, the 'golden mean'. As a practitioner, for example, it means finding the golden mean between being extremely sensitive and extremely insensitive to the needs of the client. A virtue ethics approach would hold that clients ought to be told the truth about their condition, not to maximise utility or because clients have a right to know, but because truthfulness is a virtue.

An ethic of care

Feminism and other disciplines have critiqued the adequacy of deductive, universal principles as being inadequate for describing and transforming the structural categories of social life (for example gender, race, ability and class) and for overlooking the relational aspects of social action (Tronto, 1993). A feminist ethics of care advocated by Joan Tronto (p. 60) considers 'the everyday judgements involved in activities of caring for ourselves and others'. Such a framework:

- values caring and interdependence, rather than independence, self-sufficiency and individualism;
- considers uneven power relations that are morally significant;
- attends closely to the recipients of care, thus providing a way of respecting and dealing justly with others (Held, 2011).

Care is viewed as an action and practice, rather than adherence to principles or rules, and caring allows us to live in the world as well as possible. Good care depends on the values of people engaged in caring. Crigger notes two limitations to an ethical theory of caring. Partiality and subjectivity could lead to decisions being made on the basis of emotional responses and preferences. A possible way to manage this is to infuse social justice or impartiality, that is, combining an ethics of care (holistic and contextual treatment) with an ethics of justice (equitable and fair treatment) in order to maintain ethical relationships (Botes, 2000; Crigger, 1997).

The question of culture and ethics

Resolving cross-cultural ethical dilemmas by applying universal rules can result in healthcare delivery that is ethnocentric, unequal or inappropriate

(Delany et al., 2013, p. 13). While this chapter has primarily focused on Western ethical approaches and the New Zealand healthcare system, there are many culturally based approaches to health ethics. Attempts at being 'culturally safe' across cultures can lead to competing or challenging ethical principles such as autonomy or truth telling (2013, p. 71). A culturally relativist position would hold that alternate behaviours and practices are acceptable and cannot be analysed or judged by anyone outside of that culture (Narruhn & Schellenberg, 2013, p. 376). There is debate over whether there are distinct cultural values or whether they are generally shared and whether variations within or between cultures are ignored or oversimplified (Delany et al., 2013, p. 71). One proposed solution is to find the middle ground between universalism and relativism, which is applying the universal with specificity.

Cultural safety as an ethical framework

Cultural safety is a relational framework focusing on the health professional/ client relationship and grounding ethical decision making in the context of care in combination with principles or theories. Each ethical situation is viewed as unique and takes into account the needs of each of the people in the situation whilst also having concern with the socio-political aspects of practice. This concern is evident in the *Code of Ethics* (New Zealand Nurses Organisation, p. 9):

> Nurses demonstrate ethical nursing practice when they advocate individually and collectively for the elimination of social inequities. Nurses address social inequities by: collaborating with other health care professionals and organisations for change in unethical health and social policies, legislation and regulations; advocating for accessible, appropriate and affordable health care services that are available to all; recognising the significance of the socio-economic determinants of health; and supporting environmental preservation and restoration.

Cultural safety offers practitioners an approach to practising ethically. It assumes that it is not possible to fully understand a client's culture but instead requires professionals to carefully consider the impact of their own cultural history and experience, and how this might impact on the patient's cultural practices. Such an approach assumes that the professional is not yet a fully competent cultural practitioner and is beginning from a position of limited awareness (Woods, 2010, p. 716). A fundamental tenet of cultural safety is the attention that is paid to the culture of health, which provides the framework for ethical decisions to take place.

Cultural safety has an explicit moral rationale. It assumes that safe care requires trust, which leads to greater openness and better care, which in turn can also counter healthcare inequities (Ornelas, 2008, p. 187). Having a culturally safe healthcare organisation helps to create an ethical organisation, as intercultural experience fundamentally requires attention to the 'other' which is at the heart of ethics. Attempting to eliminate racial inequities or addressing the causes of unequal care will be inadequate unless how whiteness contributes to these inequities is considered and diverse perspectives are valued (Stone, 2008, p. 222).

Cultural safety heavily emphasises the relational and recognises that health professionals[2] are culture bearers whose relationships are suffused with power. A culturally safe professional recognises that biomedicine, in combination with colonialism, are privileged so that Western approaches are considered superior to non-Western ones (Varcoe, Browne & Cender, 2014). They scrutinise the values and assumptions of the culture of health care and are aware that some moral decisions are privileged over others (Narruhn & Schellenberg, 2013, p. 377). They work to cultivate mechanisms that enable better health outcomes and equitable treatment for those marginalised by the culture of care.

It is important for professionals to be aware of the impact of culture on health and for them to use effective strategies for negotiating these differences (Delany et al., 2013, p. 12). While cultural competence is a mandatory requirement, ethical practice requires understanding the ethical implications of cultural practices rather than following rules. Using cultural safety as a starting point for resolving ethical issues requires being aware of the validity of differing world views (Narruhn & Schellenberg, 2013). Following this is the attempt to respect or accommodate a client and their family's cultural preferences, while carefully negotiating and scrutinising our own deeply held beliefs (Delany et al., 2013, p. 12). Having an analytical framework which is cognisant of the social, historical, political, institutional and economic context of health care for

---

[2] Cultural diversity is the norm rather than the exception; every health interaction is cross-cultural (Delany et al., 2013, p. 11). As the workforce is diverse, it is important to note that culture does not just refer to those receiving care who are culturally different to ourselves. Increasingly, practitioners are multicultural rather than a homogenous white service provider (Turner 2003, p. 103). Furthermore, ethical conflicts and tensions might occur within people from the same communities or language groups.

ethnic and indigenous recipients means that health professionals will be in a better position to intervene in exclusionary structural processes (Narruhn & Schellenberg, 2013, p. 377).

The following list summarises what questions a health professional needs to consider when forming an analytical framework:

1 What are the ethical issues at stake?
2 What further information do I need to gain a better understanding of the situation?
3 Are my values and frame of reference the only ones which warrant overriding consideration in this relationship?
4 How do I know that my judgements in this relationship are morally and culturally appropriate?
5 Is it possible to develop a shared understanding of the problems and hear the perspectives of all concerned?
6 What are the diverse options for addressing the situation?
7 What are the pros and cons of each option?
8 What choices can everyone live with?
9 How can the decision/action be communicated in respectful and empathetic ways?

(Points 3 and 4 are adapted from Kanitsaki, 1989, cited in Johnstone & Kanitsaki, 2009, p. 91, and the remainder are from Holstein, 2001.)

Conclusion

Ethical questions arise during everyday caring activities. The values associated with rule-based ethics are important, however, resolving ethical issues in cross-cultural caring relationships requires projecting ourselves into the world of another and extending beyond reliance on principle and rule-based ethics. In order to do this, having an interpersonal capacity to maintain a trusting relationship where communication is valued is pivotal. An ethic of care and a cultural safety framework help move strategies beyond the opposition of the individual to the universal. Supplementing an ethic of care with a consideration of the social, cultural and political contexts, in which both client and carer exist, can enhance cultural safety. The authoritative weight of institutional culture and power relations in healthcare systems can curtail and marginalise the clients' individual and collective (whānau, hapu, iwi) cultural identity and autonomy. It is in committing to the ethical experience of this difference – rather than striving to impose uniformity – that paradoxically helps create universal moral systems that are responsive to lived realities of all people.

> How might your culture, religion or background affect the value you place on particular issues?
> How might your culture, religion or background advantage some clients and disadvantage others?
> What virtues do you think practitioners should have? Are there qualities that every practitioner 'should' possess? For example, caring, compassion, honesty, integrity?
> How is an ethical theory of care similar or different to other ethical theories?
> As a health professional there might be some people you care for that you clash with or have personalities that you do not like. How should you treat them as a practitioner?

FOR REFLECTION

References

Beauchamp, T. L. & Childress, J. F. (1983). *Principles of biomedical ethics* (2nd edn.) (p. 8). New York: Oxford University Press.

Beauchamp, T. L. & Childress, J. F. (2001). *Principles of biomedical ethics* (5th edn.). New York: Oxford University Press.

Botes, A. (2000). A comparison between the ethics of justice and the ethics of care. *Journal of Advanced Nursing, 32*(5), 1071–5.

Crigger, N. J. (1997). The trouble with caring: A review of eight arguments against an ethic of care. *Journal of Professional Nursing, 13*(4), 217–21. doi:10.1016/S8755-7223(97)80091-9

Delany, C., Parker, M., Murphy, G., Guillemin, M., Hall, M. G., Fuscaldo, G. & Gillam, L. (2013). *Addressing cultural diversity in health ethics education*. Sydney: Australian Government Office of Learning and Teaching.

Doane, G. H. (2002). In the spirit of creativity: The learning and teaching of ethics in nursing. *Journal of Advanced Nursing, 39*(6), 521–8. doi:10.1046/j.1365-2648.2002.02320.x

Health and Disability Commissioner. (1996). *The HDC Code of Health and Disability Services Consumers' Rights Regulation 1996*. Retrieved 21 November 2014 from http://www.hdc.org.nz/the-act-code/the-code-of-rights/the-code-(full)

Held, V. (2011). Morality, care, and international law. *Ethics & Global Politics, 4*(3), 173–94.

Holstein, M. (2001). Bringing ethics home: A new look at ethics in the home and the community. In M. Holstein & P. Mitzen (eds) *Ethics in community-based elder care* (pp. 31–50). New York: Springer Publishing Company.

Jenkins, R. (2011). Moral imperialism. In *Encyclopaedia of global justice* (pp. 721–3). Dordrecht: Springer Publishing Company.

Johnstone, M. J. & Kanitsaki, O. (2009). Ethics and advance care planning in a culturally diverse society. *Journal of Transcultural Nursing: Official Journal of the Transcultural Nursing Society / Transcultural Nursing Society, 20*(4), 71–91. doi:10.1177/1043659609340803

Melé, D. & Sánchez-Runde, C. (2013). Cultural diversity and universal ethics in a global world. *Journal of Business Ethics, 116*(4), 681–7. doi:10.1007/s10551-013-1814-z

Narruhn, R. & Schellenberg, I. R. (2013). Caring ethics and a Somali reproductive dilemma. *Nursing Ethics, 20*(4), 366–81. doi:10.1177/0969733012453363

New Zealand Nurses Organisation. (2013). *Code of ethics.* Retrieved 21 November 2014 from http://www.nzno.org.nz/LinkClick.aspx?fileticket=pUAt5BzYuqc%3d&portalid=0

Nursing Council of New Zealand. (2012). *Code of conduct for nurses.* Retrieved 21 November 2014 from http://www.nursingcouncil.org.nz/Nurses/Code-of-Conduct

Ornelas, I. J. (2008). Cultural competency at the community level: A strategy for reducing racial and ethnic disparities. *Cambridge Quarterly of Healthcare Ethics, 17*(2), 185–94. doi:10.1017/S0963180108080213

Stone, J. R. (2008). Healthcare inequality, cross-cultural training, and bioethics: Principles and applications. *Cambridge Quarterly of Healthcare Ethics, 17*(2), 216–26. doi:10.1017/S0963180108080249

Tronto, J. C. (1993). *Moral boundaries: A political argument for an ethic of care.* London: Psychology Press.

Turner, L. (2003). Bioethics in a multicultural world: Medicine and morality in pluralistic settings. *Health Care Analysis, 11*(2), 99–117. doi:10.1023/A:1025620211852

United Nations. (1948). *Universal declaration of human rights.* Retrieved 21 November 2014 from http://www.un.org/en/documents/udhr/

Varcoe, C., Browne, A. J. & Cender, L. (2014). Promoting social justice and equity by practicing nursing to address structural inequities and structural violence. In P. N. Kagan, M. C. Smith, & P. L. Chinn (eds.) *Philosophies and practices of emancipatory nursing: Social justice as praxis.* (pp. 266–84). New York: Routledge.

Woods, M. (2010). Cultural safety and the socioethical nurse. *Nursing Ethics, 17*(6), 715–25. doi:10.1177/0969733010379296

Yarbrough, S. & Klotz, L. (2007). Incorporating cultural issues in education for ethical practice. *Nursing Ethics, 14*(4), 492–502. doi:10.1177/0969733007077883

9

Being a culturally safe researcher

Robin Kearns and Isabel Dyck

Having studied this chapter, you will be able to:

- reflect on the character of research activity;

- consider the power relations inherent in the research process;

- explore your own feelings about participating in research;

- consider what culturally safe research practice might be like.

- culture

- ethical obligations

- participant observation

Introduction

New Zealand legislation like the Health and Safety in Employment Act (1992) is aimed at ensuring that all workers, including researchers, remain physically safe. However, there has been less attention to other dimensions of the safety of researchers or the people we encounter in the course of research. An international exception is the UNESCO *Universal Declaration on Bioethics and Human Rights* (2005) which addresses the domains of medicine, life sciences and related technologies and seeks 'respect for human dignity, human rights and fundamental freedoms'. In this chapter, we reflect on the links between culture, safety and research. In particular, we consider how cultural diversity in contemporary New Zealand society requires us to consider cultural aspects of the conduct of research.

It is our contention that research involving other people should be founded on principles of partnership. Mason Durie (1988) has asserted that, following the principles of the Treaty of Waitangi, a working partnership between Māori and non-Māori will be central to the success of any Māori health research. This view has been endorsed and elaborated on in subsequent documents such as the Health Research Council of New Zealand's *Te Ara Tika: Guidelines for Māori Research Ethics* (undated). In this chapter we explore the notion of 'partnership' in research as a key element of culturally safe research and argue that Durie's assertion can, and should, inform (and even transform) social and health research in Aotearoa New Zealand – whether it involves Māori or not.

Our key argument is that culturally safe research involves three key processes:

1 respect for the cultural knowledge, values and practices of others;
2 an awareness of one's own way of seeing and doing;
3 analysis of the effect of our actions on the knowledge that is produced.

All research involves seeing the world, and seeing implies a vantage point, a place – both social and geographical – at which people position themselves to observe and be part of the world (Kearns, 2010). What is observed from this social and physical location is influenced by how people are regarded by others. A person may be seen as an 'insider' (one who belongs), an 'outsider' (one who does not belong and is 'out of place'), or as someone in between. In whatever ways researchers are perceived, critical reflection can help them to transform their research into a self-conscious, effective and ethically sound practice. This transformation can come about through recognising that as researchers they take part in the world, not just represent it (Kearns, 2010).

Making connections between culture, safety and research

Before being able to make connections between culture, safety and research, an understanding of each of these ideas needs to be developed.

Research

What, to begin with, does 'research' mean? While there are many types and purposes of research within the health and social sciences, it can be generalised by saying that all research involves sets of practices and social relationships. This fundamentally social nature of research extends into laboratory and field-based science, for even in these situations of studying inanimate objects or non-human life forms, there are relationships with others, such as co-workers or people with a vested interest in the integrity of a place (for example, local tangata whenua whose guardianship extends over the land or water being researched).

Research for those working in the social sciences and health professions can cover a wide range of approaches and topics. In this chapter, we concern ourselves with research that involves encounters with other people. This might range from simple counting exercises to closer and more sustained encounters involving multiple interactions, such as in participant observation or focus group interviews. For example, researchers might accumulate observations of pedestrians passing various points in a hospital foyer in order to establish daily rhythms of activity within healthcare institutions. In this sort of study, other elements of the immediate setting are (at least temporarily) ignored and the resulting data is easily subjected to graphical representation or statistical analysis. This is an approach to observation which may be useful for establishing trends, but ultimately it reduces experience to numbers to such an extent that any real understanding of places and their social dynamics is limited.

Most of the research conducted in the social sciences and health studies is undertaken in a more holistic manner than simply counting. Unlike laboratory-based science, it is not 'controlled' – that is, it does not concern itself only with those phenomena predetermined as significant by the researcher. A fundamental practice of research is observation and, while this refers literally to that which is seen, observation involves more than just seeing. Most obviously, it also includes listening, a critical activity of not only collecting information but also of affording dignity to the other person(s) encountered in research. Thus listening takes place in the course of techniques such as interviews and participant observation for both practical and ethical reasons.

One might argue that all research involves observation, or at least is made up of a series of observations. Thus, in a social setting, the population can 'be observed' by employing questionnaires through which the researcher establishes the frequency of certain characteristics (for example, occupation, sex or ethnicity). The activity of conducting a questionnaire survey invariably places the researcher in the position of being an 'outsider', marked as coming from another subculture by purpose, if not also by appearance and attitude. In contrast, interview research involves considerable interaction between researcher and 'researched' but, again, the researcher's positioning needs careful consideration whether as an outsider, insider or somewhere in between.

Culture

What is meant by 'culture'? Culture has a multiplicity of meanings. Not so long ago in New Zealand, culture was assumed to comprise sophisticated artistic happenings such as opera and ballet performances. At the same time there was recognition that other 'small c' cultures existed with little status and certainly no sophistication. Often their artefacts had curiosity status and lay behind glass cases in museums. Over the last few decades, this equation of 'big C' culture with the formal arts has been replaced by recognition of the diversity of cultures in our increasingly complex society.

Social scientists use the term culture to refer not just to the creative expressions of a society but also to their practices, knowledge, beliefs and sense of identity. A key point is that culture cannot be taken for granted or regarded as stable; rather is it contested (debated and argued over). Think of examples in our history in which people have protested by taking direct action: Hone Heke cutting down a pole bearing the New Zealand flag at Kororāreka (Russell) in 1844; or in 1994, Mike Smith's attack on the tree on One Tree Hill in Auckland (Kearns & Collins, 2000). These controversies invoked debate as to the appropriateness of colonial flagpoles and an iconic pine tree which, for the protagonists, symbolised a broader set of beliefs and cultural perspectives.

In the more contemporary landscape, cultural festivals often showcase the more visible aspects of culture – and not just those from other countries (for example, the Pride Festival of LGBTI cultures and the Pasifika Festival in Auckland –see Friesen, Blue & Talo, 2014). Generic 'Kiwi culture' has been celebrated in books and exhibitions, and is often associated with nostalgia for a simpler past of baches, hokey pokey ice cream and black singlets. However, ideas of any universal 'Kiwi culture' assume a broad acceptance and common histories, as well as limiting the images of non-Pākehā people and practices to stereotypes such as Māori performing haka and swinging poi.

The diversity of migrant groups that now comprise New Zealand's (especially metropolitan) population form a vibrant mix of what some might call 'subcultures'. They are based around elements such as identity, lifestyle and age. This presents a sometimes fragmented and contested image of New Zealand culture as we find it harder to define who 'Kiwis' are. Is the Asian Lantern Festival held in Auckland every February 'Kiwi culture'? Certainly not in light of tradition but possibly 'yes' when we pause to acknowledge how many New Zealand citizens with Asian heritage there are. In the 1990s, the then Prime Minister Jim Bolger once even claimed we were part of Asia! Culture certainly is not static and is constantly evolving.

Social and health research invariably brings researchers into close encounters with the questions of 'difference' and the identity politics associate with culture that prevails in contemporary New Zealand. These encounters can involve researchers realising that the difference inscribed onto their identities though bodily appearance can be a source of curiosity or even anxiety for those who they encounter (see practice example 1).

A stranger on the street

Practice example 1

While teaching a field course in research design and methods in a small regional city some years ago, one of the students of Indian descent was participating in a household survey. Such was the suspicion on the part of an older Pākehā householder that, when she saw someone with a visibly different appearance, she immediately phoned the police! The student was suddenly perturbed to notice a police car following her as she went from door to door with her clipboard and research questions.

A key responsibility for researchers is to challenge what social theorists have called 'essentialist' readings of the human condition – that is, the attribution of 'natural' characteristics such as gender, sexuality and race. These are social constructions and not merely natural phenomena that researchers must all accept.

Culture, ethnicity and race are often confused and substituted for each other in health research. Ethnicity involves self-definition on the part of individuals or groups, whereas race involves labels applied by others on the basis of observed (rather than necessarily experienced) characteristics. To elaborate with an example, the term 'Māori' was formerly used in the census in terms of 'race' given that it related to 'blood' which itself is a metaphor for parentage. In the 1990s, however, this was changed to a more ethnic use of the category that allows respondents to self-identify on the basis of affiliation and experience.

In the case of the foregoing story in practice example 1, the elderly woman, who was unaccustomed to encountering a young Indian person, had a reaction of alarm because she erroneously equated non-white skin (a perception of 'race') with a sense of threat to her security. While much discussion about cultural safety concerns the well-being of those encountered in research, in this case the researcher herself was inadvertently made to feel unsafe by the impulsive response of a potential survey respondent.

Safety

There are four dimensions of safety that are relevant to research:

1 the physical safety of researchers;
2 the physical safety of participants;
3 the emotional safety of researchers;
4 the emotional safety of participants.

These dimensions can be placed under the general 'umbrella' of cultural safety which is summarised in Table 9.1. Cell 1 signifies the physical safety of a researcher. By way of example, if a street gang known to be involved in trading illegal drugs has a reputation for violent activity, it would be foolish for a researcher to venture into undertaking field research alone on this topic. There is, first and foremost, an obligation on the part of institutions to ensure that their researchers are physically safe. Cell 2 shows the physical safety of research participants. This a particular concern in experimental medical research and drug trials. The ends (research results) can never justify

TABLE 9.1 *Dimensions of safety in research*

DIMENSION	RESEARCHERS	PARTICIPANTS
Physical safety	1	2
Emotional safety	3	4

the means (exposure of people to unsafe situations). Cell 3 is the emotional safety of a researcher. This includes not just the feelings that accompany any social interaction but also implies a sense of 'security of the self' that will be provided through respect of social differences. As in practice example 1, it is unsettling for a researcher to feel humiliated by the way they are received by others and there is a responsibility on the part of those overseeing a project to ensure, as far as possible, that people's gender, ethnicity and age are respected. This concern is among the reasons that health-related studies increasingly strive for ethnic matching of interviewers. Cell 4 has been the central focus for cultural safety concerns within the research process, with commentators suggesting that only researchers well versed in a population's historical experience and contemporary status should engage with members on matters pertaining to health. The risk is that traces of oppression embedded in social and economic structures are unintentionally endorsed by a researcher. This endorsement could be implicitly conveyed through their dress (for example, looking 'corporate' among working-class respondents), language (for example, mispronouncing Māori place names) or attitude (for example, generally being condescending towards people's circumstances) (Dyck & Kearns, 1995). One solution posed by Wilson & Neville (2009) is that research involving vulnerable populations should be designed with the involvement of group members themselves.

The foregoing discussion has assumed that safety concerns are only relevant when the two parties involved in research are in direct contact. However, the safety question can also be categorised into two time periods: *after* as well as *during* the research encounter. An example of a lack of physical safety after a research involvement could be side effects from participating in a drug trial. But, with concerns being health and social (rather than medical) research, it is more relevant to consider the emotional safety dimension. Here consider the feelings of betrayal and subsequent mistrust of researchers that could be generated by a student being confidentially told aspects of a family's history, but which subsequently are divulged in a publically available thesis. For the whānau involved, participating in any subsequent research may well feel emotionally unsafe. Indeed, if the students were, for instance, Pākehā and the family Māori, the betrayal of trust could well play into stereotypes of culturally insensitive 'Western' academics, whose interest in research is more for the good of their careers than for the good of the community.

Post-research safety issues could also be extended to include dynamics within the research community. An example might be the graduate student who completes a thesis and whose supervisor then publishes a paper in an academic journal using the student's findings without consultation and consigning her to second authorship. These examples might be called 'post-research exploitation'.

> ❯ What comes to mind when the term 'research' is mentioned?
> ❯ Have you ever undertaken some research, or set about to investigate an issue, through talking to people you have never previously met? If so, how did you feel?
> ❯ What might you expect if you were a participant in research? How might you feel?

Power

Researchers cannot usually observe directly without being present, and bodily presence brings with it personal characteristics such as race, sex and age. Belonging to dominant groups in society can mean that they potentially carry with them the power dynamics linked to such affiliations. Being a white, adult male, for instance, will invariably create challenges to being a participant in a group whose members do not share those characteristics such as a new mothers' support group. In other words, our difference in terms of key markers of societal power (or lack thereof) contributes to how able we are to be 'insiders' and participants in the quest to understand the social relations of the world around us.

More subtle challenges may be generated by level of education and the fact that some researchers are affiliated to universities. In undertaking university-based research, institutional dynamics can be carried into their acts of observing through subtle forms of social control. As they are based in, and representative of, academic institutions, it is imperative that researchers be aware of the ways in which other peoples' behaviour may be modified by their presence (Dyck & Kearns 1995).

The ways in which a researcher is perceived by those they encounter in a research situation will determine, to a large extent, the ease with which they will interact with and incorporate the researcher into their place. Embedded within the word 'incorporate' is 'corpus', the Latin word for body. The idea of 'incorporation' helps to focus on the researcher's embodiment, and to recognise that researchers take more than intentions and notebooks into any situation. They take their bodies also (Kearns, 2010). The way they clothe themselves, for instance, can be a key marker of who they are, or who they wish to be seen as, in the field.

Dressed for dialogue

While researching the inner-city experiences of psychiatric patients, Robin chose to wear older clothes to drop-in centres in order to minimise being regarded as yet another health professional or social worker intruding on patients' lives. Being a student at the time, it was easy to find place-appropriate clothes. But would blending in have been so easy if there had been an attempt to study an elite social group (for example, the dynamics at a medical specialists' convention). It is generally easier to dress 'down' than 'up' and this, to some extent, explains in small part why participant observation is more often used in studies of people less powerful than the researchers themselves (Kearns, 2010).

Ethical obligations

In institutions like healthcare organisations and universities, ethics committees have been established to be adjudicators of appropriate conduct by researchers. Instances of poor judgement on the part of researchers such as the so-called 'unfortunate experiment' at National Women's Hospital in the 1980s led to their formation in New Zealand. These committees invariably include members who are 'lay' (or general public) representatives to ensure that the views of non-researchers are heard and taken into account. It is also significant that, at least at the University of Auckland, the name of the committee was changed in 2003 from being concerned with 'human subjects' to 'human participants'. This change reflects the two-way culturally safe relations that are increasingly expected of university researchers.

Where research requires 'involvement' (a degree of participant observation), it might be argued that there is an ethical imperative to maintain contact with the community concerned. This imperative may be formalised by the requirements of university ethics committees but the stronger influence should surely come from the researcher, especially if relationships have been deepened (or restored) through the research process. As Maria Ponga noted in her study of the restoration of a marae at her turangawaewae on the East Coast, 'there is a social responsibility to carry on the ties . . . . . as we are all whānau, this has also had an added dimension of maintaining the family ties' (1998, p. 54). Such obligations may be taken for granted when pre-existing ties are involved but require careful consideration when social situations are entered into, or generated, for the sake of research.

Implications of culturally safe research

What might it mean to link the terms culture, safety and research? An openness to the cultural contexts of research can lead researchers to rethink their ways of knowing. Though the ideas emerged from, and are politically tied to, the bicultural contexts of health care in Aotearoa New Zealand, cultural safety ideas have implications for conducting research in plural societies more generally.

To be culturally safe in research is to enter a partnership with another person or members of a population group and allow them to participate in co-creating a deeper understanding of their world (see practice example 3). Applying the principles of cultural safety to research practice is more clearly evident in bicultural contexts when the two-way relationship that pervades research (the researched/researcher) is echoed within society at large (when Pākehā/Māori becomes a contemporary expression of the earlier binary construct of the coloniser/colonised). However, New Zealand is in an increasingly multicultural context in which identities are being redefined and social difference is becoming more complex.

Being culturally safe in a multicultural setting

Practice example 3

The experiences of marginalised Pacific households can easily be obscured by survey-based research designs. In a study by Cheer, Kearns and Murphy (2002), a 'window' into the links between food, poverty and housing costs was gained because the research was considered to be a priority by the community. This opened the door to supportive and ethnically matched Samoan and Cook Island 'mentors' offering to help. These people were able to recruit participants and generate dialogue with them in the presence of the (Pākehā) researcher. Just prior to our study, an article in Auckland's daily newspaper was headlined '"Leave us alone", say Otara Lab rats', in reference to the way Pacific people in Otara considered themselves over-researched. Because our study was commissioned by, and undertaken for, Otara people, it succeeded in difficult ethical terrain where other researchers had recently been ushered away.

Practising culturally safe research

To conduct culturally safe research, one must consider a number of dimensions of the research context. A key understanding is that the power dynamics brought to a research encounter may be expressed not only in the researcher's status and education, but also with those less visible and historically constructed forms of oppression that are invoked by the researcher's ethnicity, class or gender.

In light of these concerns, there are at least two possible courses of action. First, there might be an attempt to give full credence to the other cultures encountered in research in terms of their histories, beliefs and practices. Alternatively, research might only be undertaken within the confines of the researchers' own culture. Clearly, the former is the preferable path if they are to extend their horizons and become more informed citizens as well as adventurous investigators. Yet there is also merit in the latter move where, in any one project, there can be parallel studies involving people (both researchers and participants) of common ethnicity, gender or other marker of difference.

What are the barriers to 'culturally safe research practice'? First, the 'detachment' of conventional (positivist-inspired) social science can be an obstacle. In this approach, there is little room for the subtleties of culture and the propensity to enumerate can easily reduce the nuanced meanings of another ethnic group to a mere statistic. Another barrier to culturally safe research practice is only allowing academics to design, and judge the ethics of, research. There is surely a worthwhile risk to be taken in allowing community representatives to 'vet' a research proposal and even comment on its ethical dimensions.

A third barrier is the propensity of researchers to keep the results of research to themselves. Far more promises of 'feeding back' results are made than are kept. Culturally safe research requires a radical commitment to reciprocity such that ownership of results is shared and local communities can be offered ways of using the findings in their own development.

Three actions might contribute to 'the promotion of culturally safe research'. First, people can be encountered on their 'home turf'. Research engagement within community environments is likely to bring researchers a better appreciation of how people live and see their world (see practice example 4). Second, there is a need for a movement in their methodologies away from approaches that can objectify respondents. Culturally safe research promotes the dignity of others, replacing an 'us and them' dynamic with what philosopher Martin Buber calls an 'I and thou' relationship. Third, an environment of cultural safety in health research is being implicitly encouraged by the heightened emphasis on the 'consumer' and community representation in healthcare policy in general, and Primary Health Organisations, in particular.

Culturally safe observational research

Practice example 4

My embodiment as researcher was central to the culturally safe construction of knowledge about health care in Hokianga. Within the waiting area of one of the community clinics, I positioned myself with the aim of being neither an ominous presence (and thus inhibit conversation by gazing at others) nor overly welcoming of conversational engagement (hence my 'hiding' behind a newspaper). Such an arrangement was bound to break down, and did. On one occasion two locals offered to help with the crossword puzzle I was half-heartedly completing and, on another, a *kuia* entered, kissed and welcomed all present to 'her' clinic, including myself. My presence within the observed arena of social interaction thus dissolved the researcher/researched divide (from Kearns, 1997).

Conclusion

An ethic of cultural safety is paramount if researchers take seriously the potential to occupy the powerful position of constructing knowledge and mediating the experiences of research subjects. The challenge is to create conditions in which 'consumer views' occupy a place of legitimate (rather than 'alternative' or 'lesser') knowledge alongside other representations of complex social relations.

Cultural safety acknowledges that the taken-for-granted character aspects of interactions within health care and research (and, specifically, health research) need to be unveiled and their power-laden nature exposed. It also recognises that colonial history and the economic policies that have prevailed are both involved in the social production of health and access to health resources. Through these perspectives, cultural safety ideas point towards reflecting carefully on research practices, for neither methods nor language in research practice are 'innocent'. Rather they can reflect culturally based assumptions about how the world works and these assumptions are invariably anchored in the world views of the dominant population group(s) in society.

Culturally safe research is ethically sound and designed in a manner that is appropriate to the cultural contexts of its conduct. It is research that self-consciously recognises that it is inherently political through: (a) offering a methodological and analytical challenge to conventional positivist social science; and (b) contributing to the conditions necessary for positive social change. Researchers cannot be separate from those they study. They therefore need to design research that, to paraphrase the feminist theorist Trinh Minh-ha, fosters situations of 'us' speaking *with* them, rather than *about* 'them'.

References

Buber, M. (1966). *I and Thou*. Edinburgh: T & T Clark.

Cheer, T., Kearns & Murphy, L. (2002). Housing policy, poverty and culture: 'Discounting' decisions among Pacific peoples in Auckland, New Zealand. *Environment and Planning C: Government and Policy, 20*, 497–516.

Durie, M. (1988). *Whaiora: Māori health development*. Auckland: Oxford University Press.

Dyck, I. & Kearns, R. (1995). Transforming the relations of research: Towards culturally safe geographies of health and healin'. *Health and Place, 1*, 137–47.

Friesen, W., Blue, L. & Talo, R. (2014). Pasifika festival representations and realities for the wellbeing of Pacific Peoples in Aotearoa/New Zealand. In G. Andrews, P. Kingsbury & R. Kearns (eds) *Soundscapes of wellbeing in popular music* (pp. 123–44). Farnham: Ashgate Press.

Health Research Council of New Zealand (undated). *Te Ara Tika. Guidelines for Māori research ethics: A framework for researchers and ethics committee members*. Retrieved 10 September 2014 from http://www.hrc.govt.nz/sites/default/files/Te%20Ara%20Tika%20Guidelines%20for%20Mā ori%20Research%20Ethics.pdf

Kearns, R. A. (1997). Constructing (bi)cultural geographies: Research on and with people of the Hokianga District. *New Zealand Geographer, 53*(2), 3–8.

Kearns, R. A. (2010). Seeing with clarity: Undertaking observational research. In I. Hay (ed.) *Qualitative research methods in human geography* (3rd edn) (pp. 241–58). New York: Oxford University Press.

Kearns, R. A. & Collins, D. C. A. (2000). Maungakiekie/One Tree Hill: Contesting the iconography of an Auckland Landscape. *Australian-Canadian Studies 18*, 173–88.

Ponga, M. (1998). I Nga ra o Mua: (Re) constructions of symbolic layers in Te Poho-o-Hinemihi Marae. Master of Arts thesis, Department of Geography, The University of Auckland.

United Nations Educational, Scientific and Cultural Organization (UNESCO) (2005). *Universal Declaration on Bioethics and Human Rights*. Paris: UNESCO. Retrieved 10 September 2014 from http://unesdoc.unesco.org/images/0014/001461/146180E.pdf

Wilson, D. & Neville, S. (2009). Culturally safe research with vulnerable populations. *Contemporary Nurse: A Journal for the Australian Nursing Profession, 33*(1), 69–79.

part 3

Fields of
practice

10

Child, youth and family health care

Ruth Crawford

Introduction

The major focus of my nursing practice has been in child and family care in the acute hospital child health setting, adolescent and adult alcohol services and drug rehabilitation. Coupled with my research in the area of nurses' understanding of parenting in hospital, and nurses' and parents' emotional communication in hospital, I have developed a firm resolve that health professionals must have a working knowledge of culturally safe practice. Nowhere is this more critical than in the care of the child, youth and family. In this chapter, the concept of cultural safety as it relates to child, youth and family health is explored. As a Pākehā, I am aware of ways the health system in New Zealand has benefited my culture to the detriment of others', in particular, Māori. With this in mind, the transfer of power from health professionals to families and children is contended as fundamental to this process. The ensuing discussion is from my experience and perspective, so it does not attempt to discuss another culture's perspective. Relevant statistics are examined; appropriate care plans, assessments and interventions discussed; and a tool to evaluate care provided to child, youth and families in Aotearoa New Zealand is presented.

The relationship between culture and cultural safety: definitions

One of the factors influencing the introduction of cultural safety was the changing health environment in New Zealand in the late 1980s. Following the *Cartwright Report* in 1988, there was a shift in power from the health professional to the client. According to Kearns (1997), cultural safety was one manifestation of a broader trend towards transferring power in health care. Here are the key concepts that have been identified.

- 'Culture' is described as a noun, an intrinsic part of being human. It is in us, contributes to us as people and influences all our behaviours and activities (Teekman, 1995). Culture serves two functions. First, it provides the integrative beliefs and values that give an individual a sense of identity and rules of behaviour and, second, it facilitates social integration and communication among family members (Cortis, 2003). People's cultures are intrinsic to who they are and their cultures help shape their values and behaviours.
- 'Cultural safety' refers to a way of being with other people, which encourages and celebrates difference. It is not about seeing others as different from us; rather we are different from others. It is also about us accepting others' differences and acknowledging our own background and culture. Cultural safety practice must respect the many cultures of children and families.
- 'Child poverty' is defined as children who have insufficient income or material resources to enable them to survive (Boston & Chapple, 2014). New Zealand paediatrician Innes Asher suggests that a practical definition of poverty in New Zealand is 'insufficient income for health care, including transport, doctor's fees, prescription costs, hospital parking; nutritious food; adequate housing, not crowded, damp, cold or too costly; clothing, shoes, bedding, washing and drying facilities, and education, including transport, stationery, school donations, exam fees, and school trips' (Asher, 2010).

- 'Absolute' poverty involves being deprived of one or more of life's essentials such as food, water, sanitation, shelter and basic health care (Boston & Chapple, 2014).
- 'Relative poverty' is 'living in a household whose income, when adjusted for family size and composition, is less than 50 per cent of the median income for the country in which they live' (UNICEF Innocenti Research Centre, 2012, p. 3). In New Zealand, families in relative poverty earn less than 60 per cent of the median national household income after housing costs (Ministry of Social Development, 2014).
- 'Cultural broker' is a term for a person (or group) who provides a bridge, link or mediation between groups of people (Jezewski, 1990), or a liaison between two different realms, such as the healthcare system and families who enter the system (National Centre for Cultural Competence, 2004).

The child/tamariki

In Aotearoa New Zealand, a child is defined as a 'boy or girl under the age of 14 years' (this is the legal definition under the Child, Young Persons and Their Families Act, 1989, p. 28). In every culture the child is the hope for the future, as he or she represents the next generation. In Māori society the child or mokopuna descends from a culture and history based on strong genealogical or whakapapa links and relationships.

Statistics

Child, youth and family health are of major concern in New Zealand (Craig et al., 2013a; Public Health Advisory Committee, 2010). Statistics New Zealand (2014a) estimates that: 20.4 per cent of New Zealanders are under the age of 15 years with 68 per cent of children being European/New Zealander, 23.4 per cent are Māori, 12.2 per cent are Pasifika and, increasingly in New Zealand, 22.8 per cent belong to more than one ethnic group. Compared with the European/ Pākehā population, Māori and Pasifika people have a higher proportion of children, with over one third of the Māori population and one third of the Pasifika population being under 15 years of age. By comparison, less than one quarter of the European/Pākehā population are under 15 (Statistics New Zealand, 2014b).

Statistics of the health status for the population groups in New Zealand also reveal marked differences. (An analysis of why this is the case will be given later in this chapter.)

- Tamariki Māori (Māori children) aged between 0–14 years comprise 33.8 per cent of the total Māori population in New Zealand (Statistics New Zealand, 2014b). Tamariki Māori have worse health than non-Māori children across a wide range of health indicators (Ministry of Health, 2012a; Ministry of Health, 2013).
- More tamariki Māori (34%) live in poor households compared to non-Māori children (17%) (Craig et al., 2013b).
- While there have been some gains in recent years, Māori are still at higher risk of dying before the age of 15 years than are non-Māori (Statistics New Zealand, 2014c).
- There are higher death rates for tamariki Māori for most of the major causes of death in children, including injuries and poisonings, road traffic accidents, sudden unexpected death in infancy, respiratory conditions and infectious diseases (Craig et al., 2012).
- In 2012 asthma affected one in five Māori children, Māori children were twice as likely to be obese as non-Māori children and 1.7 times more likely to have had a tooth removed in the past year as non-Māori children (Ministry of Health, 2012b).
- Potentially avoidable hospital admissions such as serious skin infections, respiratory infections, influenza and pneumonia are higher for tamariki Māori than other children (Child Poverty Action Group, 2014).

Pasifika children aged 0–14 years comprise 35.7 per cent of the total Pacific population in New Zealand (Statistics New Zealand, 2014a). Pasifika children:

- are 50 times more likely than New Zealand European children and twice as likely as tamariki Māori to be hospitalised with acute rheumatic fever (Child Poverty Action Group, 2014);
- are more overweight than other New Zealand children with one in four being obese (Ministry of Health, 2012b);
- have higher rates of acute and chronic respiratory infections, serious skin infections, and infectious diseases than other New Zealand children (Statistics New Zealand, 2014d);
- have higher rates of hearing loss and poorer oral health than other children (Ministry of Health, 2008);
- experience greater barriers to accessing primary health care (Ministry of Health, 2012b).

One of the major factors behind these child health statistics is poverty. New Zealand has high rates of poverty as a consequence of governments reducing benefits, low wages for working families, high unemployment and the global recession. Over one quarter of all New Zealand children (27%) are growing up in poverty (Child Poverty Action Group, 2014). Children from Māori, Pasifika and refugee families are more likely to be poor. Growing up in poverty means that children's families cut back on fresh fruit, vegetables and meat, do not replace worn out clothes, have less than two pairs of shoes to wear, put up with feeling cold and postpone doctor's visits because of costs (Craig et al., 2013b).

Children who have been in a low income family may be more likely to leave school without qualifications, be unemployed, have children earlier and be involved in criminal activity (The Children's Social Health Monitor New Zealand, 2010).

Implications for culturally safe practice when working with children

Nurses and health professionals need to be aware of these alarming statistics in order to address the health concerns in New Zealand. New Zealand children have particularly high rates of communicable diseases and injuries. Mortality rates are much higher for Māori and Pasifika children, and they also have higher rates of bronchiectasis, tuberculosis, rheumatic fever and serious skin infections (Pubic Health Advisory Committee, 2010). There are also inequities between different ethnicities in accessing preventative measures such as immunisation (Children and Youth in Aotearoa, 2010).

When working with children, it is vital that nurses be aware of the current social/political status of the population group that the child and family identifies with. They should also be aware of Ramsden's (1992) advice that 'nurses will be educated to not blame the victims of historical social processes, for their current plight'. The Nursing Council of New Zealand ('the Nursing Council') requires registered nurses to demonstrate competency in cultural safety. Culturally safe practice requires nurses to:

- reflect on own cultural identity and recognise the impact that personal culture has on own professional practice;
- have an understanding of self, the rights of others and legitimacy of difference to work with all people who are different from them (Nursing Council of New Zealand, 2011, p. 11).

The following practice example is typical of situations facing many parents and children in New Zealand today.

Tauea and Joseph

You are working in an acute children's ward. Tauea presents to the ward with her six-month-old baby, Joseph. Joseph has severely infected eczema. Tauea is a single parent and has four older children at home. She lives with her sister and her sister's three children. Tauea appears tired and tearful. She states that she can't cope any more with Joseph's constant crying and scratching.

> ❭ Describe the clinical situation in this practice example.
> ❭ What is your nursing assessment of the situation?
> ❭ What would the consequence of this situation have been for the nurse, Joshua and Tauea?
> ❭ What are the cultural issues in this scenario?
> ❭ Describe how you would manage this situation.

In summary, two key components are required when working with children. They are:

- cultural awareness of own culture;
- cultural sensitivity to the cultural needs of the child and significant others.

Youth/rangatahi

In New Zealand, a youth or young person is between the ages of 12 to 24 years (Ministry of Youth Development, nd, p. 6). 'Youth' can be defined as 'a period of transition from the dependence of childhood to adulthood's independence'(UNESCO, 2014).

Statistics

In New Zealand, young people between 12 and 24 make up 18 per cent of the total population (Statistics New Zealand, 2014a). Unfortunately, these statistics correlate with some of the risk-taking behaviours evident during this period of development. Statistics for this group provide the following information:

- In 2012 the total death rate was 71 deaths per 100 000. More males than females died in this age group. New Zealand had the second highest youth mortality out of 27 developed countries (after the United States) (Patton et al., 2012).
- The three major causes of unintentional injury deaths are motor vehicle injuries, poisoning and drowning (New Zealand Mortality Review Data Group, 2013).
- Rangatahi Māori have a higher mortality rate than other ethnic groups, followed by Pasifika, European and Asian (New Zealand Mortality Review Data Group, 2013).
- In 2009 New Zealand had the highest rates of youth suicide in the Organisation for Economic Cooperation and Development (OECD) accounting for one fifth of all suicides in the country (Child and Youth Mortality Review Committee, 2009). In 2011, the suicide death rate for Māori youth was over twice that of non-Māori (Ministry of Health, 2014).
- In 2011 the rates of teenage pregnancy among young Māori were approximately four times higher than those of their non-Māori peers (Marie, Fergusson & Boden, 2011).
- The leading reasons for hospital admission in rangatahi Māori are issues associated with pregnancy, delivery and the postnatal period (Ministry of Health, 2012a).
- The most common cause of hospitalisation of males is injury.

Specific risks for young people are:

- binge drinking and drug taking;
- mental illness;
- injury;
- tobacco use;
- sexually transmitted infections/unwanted pregnancies (Ministry of Health, 2002).

In 2013, the Adolescent Health Research Group from the University of Auckland released the third national survey of secondary school students

(Clark et al., 2013). This document provided national data on the health and well-being of New Zealand youth. Major findings of the document were:

- health and well-being was improving;
- there were declining numbers using substances (cigarettes, marijuana and alcohol); engaging in risky driving behaviours, and being exposed to violence and sexual coercion.
- some young people were unable to access health and dental care;
- there was inconsistent condom and contraception use;
- some were overweight or obese;
- some had significant depressive symptoms.

When considering all youth, not just those who are at school, sexually transmitted infection rates are very high. For example, in 2011 the rate of chlamydia was four times that of Australia and the United Kingdom, and double that in the United States (Morgan, Colonne & Bell, 2011).

In summary, New Zealand continues to have one of the highest rates of youth suicide in the OECD. The youth suicide rate is much higher among young men than young women, and is highest for young Māori males (Ministry of Health, 2014). New Zealand has high rates of births to teenage mothers and of sexually transmitted infections (Terry, Braun & Farvid, 2012).

Maia

Practice example 2

You are a public health nurse. You visit a local coeducational school in your area to run a health clinic. Maia, aged 13, presents to the clinic. She says that she has had unprotected sex with a friend two days ago. Maia lives with her older sister and seven other family members. She does not get on with her mother. Maia identifies herself as Māori and says she is 'worried'.

FOR REFLECTION

> What would your nursing assessment of Maia include?
> Outline key aspects of your interventions.
> To whom would you refer Maia?
> What would your follow-up involve?

Implications for culturally safe practice working with youth

Working with youth requires encouraging identification with and involvement in your own ethnic culture, as well as involvement in others. Encourage youth to meet with others of the same ethnic background and develop a support group (either in the school or community) so that they can meet on a regular basis. A key aspect of working with youth is ensuring that confidentiality is maintained, as there is strong evidence that concern about breaching their confidence is a barrier to youth accessing health care (Bagshaw, 2011; Denny et al., 2013).

An awareness of and sensitivity to their youth culture is also required. Fleming and Watson (2002) recommend the following strategies to assist with this process:

- don't assume that compliance with medical treatment is the norm;
- devote as much time and skills to achieving compliance as to other aspects of care;
- utilise a developmentally appropriate consultation process;
- educate or inform in a way that is meaningful to the client;
- overtly address motivation;
- develop a mutually acceptable treatment plan;
- utilise multiple support strategies to ensure the plan works;
- promote client autonomy while maintaining family connectedness;
- acknowledge and attend to social, psychological, cultural, sexual, educational and vocational needs in addition to medical concerns.

Family

Family can be defined as 'two or more individuals who depend on one another for emotional, physical and economical support' (Kaakinen et al., 2010, p. 5). Wright and Leahey (2000) suggest that family is who they say they are, thus moving past the traditional boundaries of limiting the family using blood, adoption and marriage. For Māori, the term 'whānau' refers to Māori who share common descent and kinship (Ministry of Social Development, 2010). Further the Taskforce on Whānau-centred Initiatives has interpreted whānau to mean a 'multi-generational collective made up of many households that are supported and strengthened by a wider network of relatives' (Ministry of Social Development, 2010, p. 13).

Statistics

The New Zealand family has changed markedly over the past 60 years. It has evolved from being nuclear and family-dominated (two parents and two children) to meeting new circumstances which are different to those of three to four decades ago. In 2006, 28 per cent of children lived in one parent families, up from 10 per cent in 1976 (Families Commission, 2014). In 2010, New Zealand had more one-parent families than any other OECD country except the United States. Māori are disproportionately represented as sole parents (Children and Youth in Aotearoa, 2010). Extended families (multigenerational kinship networks of grandparents, aunts, uncles, cousins and more distant relatives) are more common among Māori and Pasifika families than among non-Māori families (Royal Commission on Social Policy, 1988).

Families in hospital

Families with children in hospital face a variety of issues, including anxiety about their children and trying to fit into the culture of the hospital ward. Parents need ongoing support and guidance to navigate their way through their hospital journey. Parents are sometimes frustrated by a fragmented health service, practitioner behaviour and lack of information (Dickinson, Smythe & Spence, 2006).

Parents' expectations of nurses in hospital

Parents are frequently vulnerable and isolated within a hospital ward. They are away from their usual supports and in a strange environment. Parents want to regain a sense of control over their lives and also to make a person to person connection with one or two nurses (Blockley & Alterio 2008). Families want support, guidance and involvement, and for nurses to ask them how they are doing (Crawford, 2014; Sarajärvi, Haapamäki & Paavilainen, 2006).

Parental sense of self

Parents' sense of self is distorted by the hospitalisation of a child. When a child is well, parents' caring behaviour produces a predictable response. When a child is in hospital, parents do not know how their child will react to their nurturing, or what nurturing is effective. At home the parents are experts; in hospital, they feel uncertain, uninformed and confused at a time when they have to adjust to sharing the care of their child with others (Crawford, 2014).

Planning

Planning culturally safe care for the child, youth and family requires the health professional to be responsive to the needs of all members of the family. Health professionals can run the risk of expecting the family to comply with ideas and advice that could promote, maintain and/or restore health. Families from different cultures are sometimes labelled difficult or problematic because of perceived lack of adherence to health professionals' desired behaviours. In reality, families may not be aware of what is appropriate behaviour in healthcare interactions which can result in misunderstandings and conflict (Coyne, 2006–07). To minimise this risk, nurses need to be in constant communication with the family so that they don't assume that their planned intervention automatically receives the 'blessing' of the family concerned.

Nurses as cultural brokers

Families wait for nurses to take the lead in the provision of care to the child and want to be involved in the child's care. They look to nurses to be a contact between them and the hospital system, a cultural broker, defined by the National Centre for Cultural Competence (2004) as a liaison between two groups. Nurses are ideally placed to provide cultural brokerage as they have understanding of some of the stresses and difficulties parents and families experience in hospital, and implicit knowledge of the ward culture (Crawford, 2014).

Communication

The way in which nurses communicate with patients and their families is central to the provision of nursing care. The culturally safe nurse will possess a range of communication skills to facilitate this process. A clear understanding of one's own culture will also prevent the assumption that families have the same values and beliefs as the nurse. In order to gauge any differences and avoid stereotyping, a cultural assessment may assist the nurse to develop a comprehensive picture of the family.

A study was carried out to describe the beliefs and self-reported practices of paediatric nurses from four children's hospitals, regarding the process of assessing culture (Hart, 1999). Five hundred and eighty-four respondents indicated that they worked in a culturally diverse population and frequently experienced cultural conflicts. Findings confirmed that cultural assessments were not routinely performed as part of the general assessment of the child. Learning more about the child's culture will improve effectiveness of nursing care. The nurse may need to consult with key people (such as Māori and Pasifika liaison) to undertake a cultural assessment, especially if the family is from a different ethnic background or English is another language.

Stereotyping

Stereotyping involves thinking about people as 'groups' and giving the group a number of oversimplified characteristics. Stereotypes can be useful as a quick way of processing and organising large amounts of information encountered in everyday life, but can become dangerous when there is reluctance to recognise individual difference within a group. This may result in judgements being made about the group (Stein-Parbury, 2014). Nurses need to assess each patient's preferences using a number of clues and ask questions in a culturally sensitive way (Accident Compensation Corporation, 2010).

Developing a partnership with families: a tool for evaluating care

Ramsden (1990) specified that the focus of cultural safety is on nurses becoming aware of the relationship between dominant and oppressed cultures. The end result is a genuine partnership where power is shared between groups involved in health care. Nursing has responded to the challenge of putting the client first, not the health professional. The concept of partnership requires mutual power sharing between the nurse and the client. To make power sharing possible, a nurse needs an understanding of own culture and the theory of power relationships (Egan, 1998).

When health professionals meet someone from another culture, they are most likely to think, 'that person differs from me', rather than 'I differ from that person'. The reason for this is twofold:

1 they usually only look at the world from their own perspective;
2 they are consciously trying to preserve their existing and trusted world view.

To overcome these assumptions, the nurse must first acknowledge the client as a person, which in turn involves acknowledgement of their culture (Teekman, 1995).

Sione

Practice example 3

You are a registered nurse working in an intensive care unit. Sione, aged four years, is admitted with a suspected fractured skull. With Sione are his father and paternal grandparents. The family's first language is Kiribati. When you meet the family, they appear angry and upset.

> What will your cultural assessment of this family involve?
> How will you effectively communicate with Sione's family?
> What are the cultural implications for your nursing care of Sione and his family?

FOR REFLECTION

Implications for practice

Nurses need to:

- acknowledge that parents, families and nurses have different expectations of one another's roles in the care of the hospitalised child;
- work towards bridging the gap by providing cultural brokerage, effective communication and negotiation;
- have a clear understanding about their own ethnic and cultural backgrounds, and recognise biases;
- form partnerships with families so that care can be evaluated through each phase of planning, assessment and intervention.

Conclusion

In conclusion, this chapter has provided definitions of key concepts within the area of child, youth and family health. Statistics, research and implications for practice have been examined. Child, youth and family nurses who demonstrate culturally safe practice are highly sought after in Aotearoa New Zealand and other countries throughout the world. They are accommodating and respectful of the diverse ways of being and thinking of the child, youth and family. They are open and ready to learn another way of being. All nurses have the capacity to practise in a way that is culturally safe, for themselves and for the people to whom they provide a service.

> Nurses are very powerful. We need to work with patients and families to provide care that acknowledges not only their ethnic background, but also gender, sexual orientation, occupation, religion. I don't think cultural safety is just about being/nursing Māori. (Research participant in Richardson et al., 2009, p.32)

References

Accident Compensation Corporation. (2010). *Guidelines on Māori cultural competencies for providers.* Retrieved 20 November 2014 from http://www.acc.co.nz/PRD_EXT_CSMP/groups/external_providers/documents/guide/wcm2_020645.pdf

Asher, I. (2010). The Porritt Lecture. November, Whanganui, New Zealand. Retrieved 20 November 2014 from http://www.cpag.org.nz/assets/Health/MIAsherPorrittLecture3Nov2010%20%282%29.pdf

Bagshaw, S. (2011). *Youth health enhancing the skills of primary care practitioners in caring for all young New Zealanders: A resource manual.* Christchurch: The Collaborative for Research and Training in Youth Health and Development Trust.

Blockley, C. & Alterio, M. (2008). Patients' experiences of interpersonal relationships during first time acute hospitalisation. *Nursing Praxis in New Zealand, 24*(2), 16–26.

Boston, J. & Chapple, S. (2014). *Child poverty in New Zealand.* Wellington: Bridget Williams Books Limited.

Child and Youth Mortality Review Committee, Te Ropu Arotake Auau Mate o te Hunga Tamariki, Taiohi. (2009). Fifth report to the Minister of Health: *Reporting mortality 2002–2008.* Wellington: Child and Youth Mortality Review Committee.

Child Poverty Action Group. (2014). *Our children, our choice: Priorities for policy.* Auckland: Child Poverty Action Group.

Child, Young Person and Their Families Act 1989. Retrieved 20 November 2014 from http://www.legislation.govt.nz/act/public/1989/0024.html

Children and Youth in Aotearoa. (2010). *New Zealand non-governmental organisation alternative report to the United Nations Committee on the Rights of the Child.* Auckland: Action for Children and Youth Aotearoa.

Clark, T.C., Fleming, T., Bullen, P., Denny, S., Crengle, S., Dyson, B., ... & Utter, J. (2013). Youth'12 Overview: The health and wellbeing of New Zealand secondary school students in 2012. Auckland: The University of Auckland.

Cortis, J. D. (2003). Culture, values and racism: Application to nursing. *International Nursing Review*, 55–66.

Coyne, I. (2006–07). The 'good' family syndrome: Social and cultural issues in community and family health. *Contemporary Nurse: A Journal for the Australian Nursing Profession*, 23(2), 154–6.

Craig, E., Adams, J., Oben, G., Reddington, A., Wicken, A. & Simpson, J. (2012). *Te Ohonga Ake: The health status of Māori children and young people in New Zealand.* Wellington: Ministry of Health.

Craig, E., Adams, J., Oben, G., Reddington, A., Wicken, A. & Simpson, J. (2013a). *The health status of children and young people in New Zealand.* Wellington: Ministry of Health.

Craig, E., Reddington, A., Wicken, A., Oben, G. & Simpson, J. (2013b). *Child Poverty Monitor 2013 Technical Report* (Updated 2014). Dunedin: NZ Child & Youth Epidemiology Service, University of Otago.

Crawford, R. M. (2014). *Emotional communication between nurses and parents of a child in hospital.* PhD thesis, University of Techology, Sydney.

Denny, S., Farrant, B., Cosgriff, J., Harte, M., Cameron, T., Johnson,... & Robinson, E. (2013). Forgone health care among secondary school students in New Zealand. *Journal of Primary Healthcare*, 5(1), 11–18.

Dickinson, A. R., Smythe, E. & Spence, D. (2006). Within the web: The family-practitioner relationship in the context of chronic childhood illness. *Journal of Child Health Care*, 10(4), 309–25.

Egan, J. (1998). Why has nursing adopted cultural safety as part of its preparation for practice? Beginning Journeys: A Collection of Work. Faculty of Health and Science, Christchurch Polytechnic. Retrieved 21 November 2014 from http://repository. cpit.ac.nz/eserv.php?pid=cpit:2638&dsID=BeginningJourneys_vol4_1998.pdf

Families Commission. (2014). *Families and Whānau status report 2014.* Retrieved 20 November 2014 from http://www.familiescommission.org.nz/default/files/downloads/Families-and-Whānau-Status-Report-2014.pdf

Fleming, T. & Watson, P. (2002). Enhancing compliance in adolescents: If only they'd do what they're told. *Current Therapeutics*, 43(3), 14–18.

Hart, D. (1999). Assessing culture: Paediatric nurses' beliefs and self-reported practices. *Journal of Paediatric Nursing*, 14(4), 255–62.

Jezewski, M. A. (1990). Culture brokering in migrant farmworker health care. *Western Journal of Nursing Research, 12*(4), 497–513.

Kaakinen, J. R., Gedaly-Duff, V., Coehlo, D. P. & Hanson, S. M. H. (2010). *Family health care nursing: Theory, practice and research* (4th edn.). Philadelphia: F.A. Davis Company.

Kearns, R. (1997). A place for cultural safety beyond nursing education? *The New Zealand Medical Journal, 110*(1037), 23–24.

Marie, D., Fergusson, D. M. & Boden, J. M. (2011). Cultural identity and pregnancy/parenthood by age 20: Evidence from a New Zealand birth cohort. *Social Policy Journal of New Zealand, 37*, 19–36.

Ministry of Health. (2002). *Youth health: A guide to action.* (November). Wellington: Ministry of Health.

Ministry of Health. (2008). *Pacific child health: A paper for the Pacific Health and Disability Action Plan review.* Wellington: Ministry of Health.

Ministry of Health. (2012a). *Te Ohonga Ake: The health status of Māori children and young people in New Zealand.* Wellington: Ministry of Health.

Ministry of Health. (2012b). *The health of New Zealand children 2011/12: Key findings of the New Zealand health survey.* Wellington: Ministry of Health.

Ministry of Health. (2013). *The health of Māori adults and children.* Wellington: Ministry of Health.

Ministry of Health. (2014). *Suicide facts: Deaths and intentional self-harm hospitalisations 2011.* Retrieved 20 November 2014 from http://www.health.govt.nz/publication/suicide-facts-deaths-and-intentional-self-harm-hospitalisations-2011

Ministry of Social Development. (2010). *Whānau Ora: Report of the Taskforce on Whānau-centred initiatives.* Retrieved 21 November 2014 from http://www.msd.govt.nz/documents/about-msd-and-our-work/publications-resources/planning-strategy/whānau-ora/whānau-ora-taskforce-report.pdf

Ministry of Social Development. (2014). *Household incomes in New Zealand: Trends in indicators of inequality and hardship 1982 to 2013.* Wellington: Ministry of Social Development.

Ministry of Youth Development. (nd). *An introduction and context for the development of youth policy.* Wellington: Ministry of Youth Development. Retrieved 20 November 2014 from http://www.myd.govt.nz/documents/policy-and-research/policy-document-final.pdf

Morgan, J., Colonne, C. & Bell, A. (2011). Trends of reported chlamydia infections and related complications in New Zealand, 1998–2008. *Sex Health, 8*(3), 412–18.

National Centre for Cultural Competence. (2004). *Bridging the cultural divide in health care settings: The essential role of cultural broker programs.* Georgetown: Georgetown University Centre for Child and Human Development, Georgetown University Medical Centre.

New Zealand Mortality Review Data Group. (2013). *NZ Child and Youth Mortality Review Committee: 9th data report, 2008–2012.* Retrieved 21 November from http://www.hqsc.govt.nz/assets/CYMRC/Publications/CYMRC-ninth-data-report-2008-2012.pdf

Nursing Council of New Zealand. (2011). *Guidelines for cultural safety, the Treaty of Waitangi, and Māori health in nursing, education and practice.* Wellington: Nursing Council of New Zealand.

Patton, G. C., Coffey, C., Cappa, C., Currie, D., Riley, L., Gore, F., Degenhardt, L., Richardson, D., Astone, N., Sangowawa, A. O., Mokdad, A. & Ferguson, J. (2012). Health of the world's adolescents: A synthesis of internationally comparable data. *The Lancet, 379*(9826), 1665–75.

Public Health Advisory Committee. (2010). *The best start in life: Achieving effective action on child health and wellbeing.* Wellington: Ministry of Health.

Ramsden, I. (1990). *Kawa Whakaruruhau: Cultural safety in New Zealand.* Wellington: Ministry of Education.

Ramsden, I. (1992). Teaching cultural safety. *New Zealand Nursing Journal, 85*(1), 21–3.

Richardson, S., Williams, T., Finlay, A. & Farrell, M. (2009). Senior nurses' perceptions of cultural safety in an acute clinical practice area. *Nursing Praxis in New Zealand, 25*(3), 27–36.

Royal Commission on Social Policy Te Kominhana a te Karauna mo nga ahuatanga-a-iwi. (1988). *The April Report. Volume I. New Zealand Today.* Wellington: Daphne Brasell Associates.

Sarajärvi, A., Haapamäki, M. L. & Paavilainen, W. (2006). Emotional and informational support for families during their child's illness. *International Nursing Review, 53*, 205–10.

Statistics New Zealand. (2014a). *Census Data 2013.* Wellington: Statistics New Zealand.

Statistics New Zealand. (2014b). *2013 Census QuickStats about culture and identity.* Retrieved 21 November 2014 from http://www.stats.govt.nz/Census/2013-census/profile-and-summary-reports/quickstats-culture-identity.aspx

Statistics New Zealand. (2014c). *Life expectancy and death rates.* Retrieved 20 November 2014 from http://www2.stats.govt.nz/domino/external/web/nzstories.nsf/092edeb76ed5aa6bcc256afe0081d84e/82dfd788a5ad21c1cc256b180004bacf?OpenDocument

Statistics New Zealand. (2014d). *Health and Pacific peoples in New Zealand.* Retrieved 20 November 2014 from http://www.stats.govt.nz/browse_for_stats/people_and_communities/pacific_peoples/pacific-progress-health/overall-health.aspx

Stein-Parbury, J. (2014). *Patient and person: Interpersonal skills in nursing* (5th edn.). Chatswood, NSW, Australia: Churchill Livingstone/ Elsevier.

Teekman, B. (1995). *Cultural safety: An explorative study of the concept of cultural safety in nursing.* Palmerston North: Faculty of Nursing and Health, Manawatu Polytechnic.

Terry, G., Braun, V. & Farvid, P. (2012). Structural impediments to sexual health in New Zealand: Key informant perspectives. *Sexuality Research and Social Policy,* 9(4), 317–26.

The Children's Social Health Monitor New Zealand. (2010). Retrieved 20 November 2014 from http://www.nzdoctor.co.nz/media/377444/the%20new%20zealand%20childrens%20social%20health%20monitor%202010%20advance%20embargoed%20copy.pdf

UNESCO. (2014). *Learning to live together.* Retrieved 20 November 2014 from http://www.unesco.org/new/en/social-and-human-sciences/themes/youth/youth-definition/

UNICEF Innocenti Research Centre. (2012). Measuring child poverty: New league tables of child poverty in the world's rich countries. *Innocenti Report Card 10.* Florence: UNICEF Innocenti Research Centre.

Wright, L. M. & Leahey, M. (2000). *Nurses and families: A guide to family assessment and intervention* (3rd edn.). Philadelphia: F.A. Davis Company.

11

Cultural safety in mental health A PRACTICE EXAMPLE

Fran Richardson, Rosemary McEldowney
and Thelma Puckey

Learning objectives

Having studied this chapter, you will be able to:

- critically analyse social, political, historical and cultural factors shaping healthcare relationships with people using mental health services and their whānau/family;

- demonstrate an integrated understanding of cultural safety, ethics and person-centered nursing;

- assess and evaluate contexts and influences shaping relationships with mental health patients, whānau and health professionals in mental healthcare settings;

- actively use reflection to assess, evaluate and guide safe competent person-centered care.

Key terms and concepts

- cultural safety

- *Diagnostic and Statistical Manual of Mental Disorders (DSM-5)*

- ethics

- Mental Health (Compulsory Assessment and Treatment) Act (1992)

- power

- recovery

- stigma/discrimination

- Te Tiriti o Waitangi/the Treaty of Waitangi

- trust

Introduction

The definition of cultural safety and the history of its development have been addressed elsewhere in this book. It has been established that cultural safety is about understanding the way power shapes and influences healthcare practices and healthcare outcomes for patients or clients using healthcare services. Central to the presence or absence of experiencing care as culturally safe is the degree of trust between the nurse and the patient (Ramsden, 2002). A culturally competent nurse builds a trusting environment through effective communication and considered actions.

Being competent requires the nurse to reflect on and interpret professional and institutional practices and assess how these might enhance or limit a patient's sense of safety. Culturally safe care is the subjective experience of care that is assessed as safe by the patient (Ramsden, 2002). Nurses care for people when they are at their most vulnerable and when their ability to be autonomous or in control may be compromised because of their illness or situation (Dinc & Gastmans, 2012). Trustworthiness of the nurse by the patients means that they can rely on the nurse to keep them safe from harm, hence cultural safety.

Drawing on the cultures of the nurse, the client and the setting, we provide a brief overview of mental health nursing in Aotearoa New Zealand. A practice example – Ruby's story – is then presented, interpreted and critiqued within a mental health nursing context. At the end of the chapter reflective questions are posed to guide exploration of events in the story. A framework for implementing the Te Tiriti o Waitangi/the Treaty of Waitangi ('the Treaty') in mental health concludes the chapter.

The practice example presented in this chapter is analysed and interpreted in relation to the culture of the person being cared for. The interpretation and critique of the example is shaped by our background and experience as Pākehā mental health nurses and educators. Our histories, cultures, values and beliefs position us differently from patients. We recognise that there will be different interpretations of the example and suggest that you remain open to a range of possibilities when working through the reflective activities.

Practising in a culturally safe way requires nurses to work comfortably and thoughtfully with clients whose cultures differ from their own. This means being able to reflect on and critique their own actions and interactions with clients who may be not share the same cultural or social backgrounds. Recognising 'the central place of secure cultural identity to mental health' is an important element of mental health nursing (New Zealand College of Mental Health Nurses, 2012 p. 3). The Nursing Council of New Zealand (2011) states that 'difference may include age or generation, gender, sexual orientation, occupation and socio-economic status, ethnic origin or migrant experience, religious or spiritual belief, and disability' (p. 7). While understanding that categories of difference can be helpful for a student beginning to learn about diversity, it is important to note that limiting 'difference' to set categories can mean overlooking more subtle differences that become apparent only within the complexity of everyday nursing encounters. Understanding how different variables operate within nurse–patient relationships can equip the nurse to work with complexity, uncertainty and ambiguity in everyday practice (McEldowney & Conner, 2011).

Discourses of mental health practice

There are three key discourses that have shaped and continue to shape contemporary practice: the culture of the mental health setting, the mental health nurse and the client.

Discourses or practices are ideas and thoughts reflecting a particular way of thinking within a profession or about an issue. For example, in the practice example in this chapter, discourses of medicine, nursing, historical and consumer discourses compete with one another and all impact on the person's care. Understanding the present can sometimes be helped by knowing about the past. The next section provides an historical overview of mental health nursing to provide a context.

The culture of the mental health setting

Contemporary mental health nursing has its roots in nineteenth-century health reform movements in Britain and the United States (Carpenter, 1980; Church, 1987; Dingwell, Rafferty & Webster, 1993; Jacob, Holmes & Buus, 2008; Prebble, 2007; Rush, 2004). Prior to the reforms, people with mental or psychiatric illnesses were considered to lack self-control, considered insane, immoral or criminal (Jacob, Holmes & Buus, 2008; Prebble, 2007; Rush, 2004). The reforms focused on illness, confinement and hospitalising people with mental illness as a way to provide care, treatment and protection. A thread running through these reforms was the need to maintain discipline and order through control of behaviour, morality and hygiene (Richardson & MacGibbon, 2010). The reform movements and a focus on moral treatment saw a move away from control, punishment and isolation within communities, to the establishment of large institutions where people with mental illness could be contained and the public could be protected. In the late 18th to early 20th centuries psychiatry evolved with a focus on discipline and medicalisation of behaviour. This, together with the establishment of institutions (asylums), provided a place of refuge and protection for the people with mental illnesses (Foucault, 1974; Rush, 2004). The purpose of institutional care was twofold – while it provided care and protection for the patient and provided safety for the public, it also disempowered the patient through the process of institutionalisation. Patients had little choice to be active participants in their own care. In an asylum structure, the nurse's role was one of care and protection through surveillance and observation. This was called the 'clinical gaze' (Jacob, Holmes & Buus, 2008), and included observing and reporting behaviour and the effects of treatment to determined interventions. The role included assisting with the administration of physical treatments, constraint of patients, and ensuring patient and public safety. The purpose of institutional care was twofold – the moral treatment and protection of patients paired with medical dominance to better manage psychiatric intervention .

The moral focus and the institutional structure of psychiatric nursing persisted until the 1960s where nursing work was mostly confined to large state psychiatric institutions. It was also intrinsically connected to the work of psychiatrists and the medical model of health care. This setting assumed that 'experts' – doctors and nurses – knew what was best for a person. There was little input into care from the person diagnosed with psychiatric (mental) illness. Care was delivered and received with little thought given to the patient's culture or well-being. The egalitarian ethos of treating everybody the same *regardless* of their individual culture or personal needs was a core value that permeated nursing knowledge and practice. During the 1970s and 1980s, the ideal of community treatment, as opposed to institutional care, gained momentum with more nurses working in community settings. The preference for community treatment and care was further accelerated with the advent of deinstitutionalisation and the closure of large psychiatric hospitals. Providing care to people in the community broaded the nurses' perspectives of patients and their life situations, and drew attention to the impact of socioeconomic and cultural factors on mental health and well-being. Short-stay acute mental health units were incorporated into general hospital structures and specialised units were created for people with specific mental health concerns. For example, forensic services, dual diagnosis or culturally specific units replaced structures reminiscent of the nineteenth-century asylum system.

The culture of the mental health nurse

During the 1960s and 1970s, a nursing focus on primary health care and the growing consumer movements saw further challenges to institutional models of care. This led to a shift from the use of the term 'psychiatric illness' to 'mental health/mental illness' and 'wellness'. The roles and titles of nurses working in the mental health field also changed from 'mental nurse' (1930s–mid-1940s) to 'psychiatric nurse'(mid-1940s–1970s) then to 'mental health nurse' (1980s onwards). The term 'mental health nurse' was changed in 2009 by Te Pou o Te Whakāro Nui (2009). The current title is 'mental health and addiction nurse'. For the purposes of this chapter we refer to the nurse as being a 'mental health nurse'.

Mental health nursing is a specialised area of nursing practice focusing on promoting health through assessment, clinical judgement diagnosis and treatment of people diagnosed with mental illness. The therapeutic use of self is the process through which these activities are managed; hence the defining characteristic of mental health nursing is often identified as the therapeutic relationship. Contemporary mental health nursing claims a therapeutic interpersonal relationship as being central to the work of mental health nursing (Cutliffe & Happell, 2009; Horsfall, Stuhmiller & Champ, 2000).

Hildegarde Peplau (Callaway, 2002) and Joyce Travelbee (Peplau, 1952; 1994; Travelbee, 1971) were early advocates of the therapeutic relationship as a core skill of mental health nursing. Peplau's (1952) therapeutic relationship model shifted the focus of nursing away from treating everyone the same to looking at the interpersonal nature of the relationship between the nurse and the patient. Similarly, cultural safety saw a shift away from treating everybody *regardless* of culture to treating people *with regard* to their culture (Ramdsen, 2002). Recognition of the centrality of the therapeutic relationship, together with deinstitutionalisation and other changes, shifted nursing from service-based models of care to more person-centred approaches. Mental health nurses were free to explore different approaches and models of nursing intervention. Group therapy and training, such as gestalt, psychodrama, psychoanalysis, cognitive behaviour therapy and behaviour modification, opened up new ways of thinking about illness, health and nurse–client relationships.

Nevertheless, the roles of observer, assessor and recorder of patient behaviour, 'giver of treatment', and 'provider of safety and protection' are still integral to nursing practice. Such roles give rise to tensions and complexities that the mental health nurse has to negotiate and navigate to provide safe person-centered culturally safe care (Barker, 2001; Ramsden, 2000; 2002).

The culture of the client

Coinciding with the process of deinstitutionalisation in the 1980s and 1990s, marginalised individuals and groups in society at large (such as women, indigenous groups, physically and mentally disabled people, gays and lesbians) were demanding change to traditional power structures. They sought visibility and inclusion in decision-making processes in dominant institutions (for example, health, educational and judicial), particularly as it related to them. Two such challenges occurred in Aotearoa New Zealand. One challenge arose from mental health patients who wanted their experience of mental illness and treatment to be taken into account during the process of care and treatment (Deegan, 1992; Barker, 2001; Rush, 2004). Another challenge came from Māori nurses who expressed the urgent need for mainstream health and education policy makers to address inequities in the delivery of health care and education programmes for Māori and students using health and education services (Ramdsen, 2002). These and other challenges to dominant practices, for example, the flattening of traditional hierarchies within mental health governance structures and a growing community-focused mental health structure, influenced changes in mental health practice for health professionals and the development of cultural safety. Cultural safety challenged the power inherent in the health professionals' role in mental health (Cutliffe & Happell, 2009; Ramsden, 2002).

In earlier times 'insane' or 'criminally insane' people were removed from society for the protection of the public. With the advent of more enlightened mental health practices and legislation, enlightened social attitudes followed. After years of education and development of more liberal thinking, and considerable research evidence, there still remains deep-seated stigma and discrimination towards people living with a mental illness. Stigma and discrimination can cause stress for these people as well as for their families. As a result, stigma can impact negatively on recovery and well-being (Horsfall, Cleary & Hunt, 2010; Bradley & De Souza, 2013). This brings us to Ruby's story.

Ruby's story

The context of this story identifies themes that are similar in other mental health stories that nurses may encounter in practice. The story is a fictionalised account highlighting issues of power, relationship, identity, vulnerability, and trust, duty of care, stigma, ethics and socio-political complexity. These concepts are explored in the context of the cultures of the setting, the client and the nurse.

Since 1992, cultural safety has been an inherent part of the undergraduate nursing curricula in Aotearoa New Zealand. Registered nurses are required to demonstrate culturally safe practice in various domains of competence (Nursing Council of New Zealand, 2005/2011). Māori experience of health services provided an impetus for cultural safety and nowhere is its implementation more critical than in the area of Māori mental health. Māori continue to be over-represented as consumers of mental health services, and mental health problems remain a major concern (Durie & Te Kingi, 1997; Reid, Robson & Jones, 2000). Wilson (2008) found that health and well-being influence Māori womens' health outcomes over time. Māori women understand health as being wholistic, culturally, socially and individually determined. This experience of self can create tensions when seen alongside the biomedical model, which tends to focus on ill health, and reduces people to diagnostic diagnostic categories as listed in the *Diagnostic and Statistical Manual of Mental Disorders* (DSM-5) (American Psychiatric Association, 2013).

As you read the following practice example, keep in mind your thoughts, feelings and responses to Ruby's story and the situation in which she finds herself. At the end of this story you will be asked to think about her experience and that of the nurse. The process of reflecting will provide ideas, questions and possible resolutions or solutions to the situation.

Ruby's story

Practice example

One afternoon, Ruby, a 55-year-old Māori woman is admitted informally to an acute in-patient mental health unit in a city hospital. She is accompanied by her daughter, Kiri, and son, Ruben. This is not Ruby's first admission and she is comfortable with people using her first name. Ruby has a diagnosis of bipolar affective disorder as described in the DSM-5 (American Psychiatric Association, 2013). Ruby is a valued and active member of her community and enjoys looking after her mokopuna (grandchildren). Her current behaviour is out of keeping. For the past few weeks Ruby has not been sleeping and has not been taking her prescribed medication. In the last few days she has been drinking alcohol excessively and engaging in arbitrary, random and unsafe sexual activity. Following an initial assessment, the community mental health team (CMHT) liaises with the mental health service access coordinator. Arrangements are made with Ruby and her whānau for her to go to a crisis respite house for the weekend where she can take her medication regularly thus reducing any need for admission. Ruby walks out of the respite house during the night and, following further discussion with the CMHT, it is decided to admit Ruby informally to the mental health unit for further assessment and treatment.

On admission, Ruby is in a highly agitated state – she is irritable and impatient. She does not want to be in the unit and is particularly fearful of being 'locked up' in the intensive care area (ICA). Her daughter and son want Ruby to be admitted. They believe that she needs to be somewhere safe from the potential harm associated with her behaviour. People in her community are also starting to talk about her, saying 'She's mad and dangerous'. At this stage they are unable to provide the care that they think she needs. Ruben is trying to calm his mother and get her to stay in the unit. Ruby is resisting his attempts. Kiri also tries to calm her mother and says 'you need to stay here Mum and get well'. 'You know Cindy'. Cindy, the nurse admitting Ruby, has cared for her on previous admissions and knows her and the whānau well.

Cindy undertakes a nursing assessment with Ruby and her son and daughter, with Ruby's permission. It includes questions such as:

> Will any other whānau (family) come to visit?

> Will anybody be staying with Ruby in the unit or nearby?

> Would you like the Kaimanāki (Māori support person) contacted?

> How have you been managing the changes in Ruby's behaviour over the past few weeks/days?

Cindy undertakes a risk assessment to establish Ruby's risk of causing harm to herself or others. Kiri and Ruben express concern about their mother's high risk-taking behaviour since she has been in a manic state. They comment that it would be dreadful if their mother knew what she had been doing and would be deeply ashamed. Cindy shares her own concerns regarding the potential for Ruby to impulsively leave the unit, and engage in further risk-taking behaviours. There have been similar incidents of this during previous admissions, which escalated her condition and meant that she had to be admitted to the ICA for her own safety.

The following day, Ruby *does* leave the unit without telling anyone where she is going and cannot be located. Three days later, she is found in a motel unit by a nurse from the CMHT. Ruby is partly clothed, incoherent and smells strongly of alcohol. Her manic state has escalated further. When Ruby returns to the in-patient unit, she continues to loudly express not wanting to be 'sent to the lock-up' (ICA). However, Kiri and Ruben are adamant that she should be in a safe environment and be contained to prevent any further incidents. This means that she will have to be sectioned under the Mental Health (Compulsory Assessment and Treatment) Act ('the Act') (1992). The Kaimanāki and Cindy are supportive of the position of whānau and are also aware of Ruby's not wanting to be in the ICA. Ruby's situation is discussed at a multidisciplinary treatment team meeting where a team member considers it a breach of Ruby's human rights to be contained under the Act. The staff member thinks that containment is inconsistent with providing treatment in the least restrictive manner according to the Act. He maintains that her behaviour can be managed in the unit with increased observation and medication. The outcome of this meeting is that Ruby's admission status remains informal and, as a consequence, she continues to absent herself from the unit, continues with her high risk-taking behaviour and becomes increasingly unwell. Ruby's whānau are very distressed that she hasn't stayed in the unit and that her pattern of behaviour has continued. They ask for a second clinical opinion and decide to lay an official complaint with the patient advocate. The outcome of the complaint results in Ruby being 'sectioned' under the Act and admitted to the ICA. What happens next?

Interpretation and critique of the story

Ruby's is one among many similar stories. It highlights the complexity of mental health nursing practice and draws out some key cultural safety issues that are present in everyday practice. Some of the underlying premises of cultural safety include understanding personal, professional and institutional power, and how these impact on the nurse–patient relationship and healthcare delivery.

With this background in mind, consider what needs to be taken into account when reflecting on the experience of Cindy and Ruby as they negotiate their way through Ruby's current situation. Think about:

> the provision of health care that might enable Ruby to have some control and power over her situation;

> her physical, social, emotional and cultural safety, and the effect of stigma on her recovery;

> help for her and her whānau so that they can regain full autonomy over their lives and relationships, and the values and beliefs of the health professionals in this setting.

Ruby's situation presents several tensions that Cindy has to address in establishing a therapeutic relationship. On the one hand, there is a need for Cindy to deliver care within a biomedical framework in order to meet professional and legislative requirements such as the use of the DSM-5 and the Act. She also needs to understand a recovery approach (Blueprint, 2012; O'Hagan, 2001). On the other hand, Cindy is working within a nursing framework (New Zealand College of Mental Health Nurses, 2012; Nursing Council of New Zealand, 2005/2011), where both recognise the dual roles of caring and healing inherent in the therapeutic relationship, and the need for protection through containment. Biomedical, consumer-focused recovery and nursing frameworks coexist. They work in tandem in everyday mental health practice. It is important, therefore, that mental health nurses are able to critique the underlying assumptions inherent in each framework so that one does not take precedence over another (Horsfall, Stuhlmiller & Champ, 2000). Furthermore, Cindy's practice is informed by the principles of cultural safety, which address the impact of power on the therapeutic relationship, thus adding another dimension to Ruby's care.

Cindy is working with a number of powerful competing discourses including identity, consumer participation, nursing, medice, history and cultural influences. Note that, within a shared multidisciplinary team context, these discourses are more likely to be made visible as team members express their views on what might be happening and what needs to happen for Ruby. Different discourses may influence Cindy at different times depending on how she sees herself in the situation. This in turn will shape her assessment and decision making. The story suggests that Cindy's assessment of Ruby is that she needs to be in a protected environment such as the ICA, which would mean invoking the Act and changing her patient status from informal to formal. She should be mindful that practising in a culturally safe way means protecting Ruby's personal and cultural integrity and well-being (Ramsden, 2002), as well as creating an environment of trust where Ruby can have as much autonomy as her situation allows.

> What are your initial thoughts and feelings about what is happening?
> What events or factors might be influencing Cindy's assessment of Ruby?
> What is it about Ruby's situation that might lead to her being detained under the Act?
> What factors does Cindy need to consider when providing care and protection for Ruby?
> How might Cindy work with the whānau when making decisions about Ruby's care?
> Identify at least two discourses influencing the current situation.
> How might these enable or constrain Ruby's care and treatment?

Practice example continued

Ruby has been admitted because of her seriously disturbed mental state and associated behavioural risks – she has not been sleeping or taking prescribed medication. She has been drinking alcohol excessively, and engaging in random, unsafe and unprotected sexual activity. Ruby's mental state, resultant behaviour and distress are compromising her ability to meet her survival, safety and everyday needs. She is vulnerable because of her mental state, therefore the possibility of her having control (or sovereignty) over her life or situation is compromised. Cindy must consider what Ruby needs in order for her to have control over her situation and what may impede Ruby achieving this.

Ruby is agitated, irritable and impatient, and expresses fear about being *locked up*. She is not in full control of her life or her situation. Having cared for Ruby before, Cindy knows that Ruby's behaviour will stabilise if she has a safe, protected space where this can happen. In the past, Ruby has been contained in the ICA where she has settled after a few days. Watkins (2001) cites a United Kingdom study in which mental health clients identified needs and wants when in distress. Some of these included: being able to talk to someone; being helped to manage feelings of distress; being supported by someone who listens; being helped to relax; having somewhere to be safe and cared for when unwell. Further, Grant (2003, p. 525) notes that people 'admitted on a voluntary basis often experience the admission as coercive with many subsequently attempting to leave, only to be compulsory admitted to prevent them from doing so'.

> What might be contributing to Ruby's fear and anxiety about being 'locked up'?
> Are there alternatives to containment in an ICA that would meet Ruby's needs but at the same time protect her from the consequences of her disinhibited behaviour?
> How could Cindy provide an environment for Ruby to feel less fearful and anxious?

FOR REFLECTION

Cindy can engage with Ruby in her distressed state by working closely with her and her whānau to reduce her fear and anxiety. Most importantly for culturally safe and therapeutic practice, Cindy can work to help create a supportive and trusting environment where Ruby can feel valued, respected and heard. Conversely, as a registered nurse, Cindy also has the authoritative power to detain and contain Ruby under Section 111 of the Act. This might create tension for Cindy as she strives to provide culturally safe care within a legislative framework. Cindy may be perceived by Ruby as having power over her even though she is not a stranger to her.

Cultural safety in mental health nursing

It is recognised that people's experience of mental distress will be influenced by culture. While this is a given, it should be noted that there is diversity within contemporary cultures. 'It cannot be assumed that all members of a particular culture subscribe to a particular view of that culture' (O'Brien & Morrison-Ngatai, 2003, p. 534). Ruby's culture *is* central to her identity – her family has said that her 'behaviour is not consistent with her usual way of being. She is a valued and active member of her iwi (tribe) and hapū (subtribe)'. Ruby is known as having a long history of contact with mental health services and a diagnosis of bipolar affective disorder. Therefore she has been observed, assessed and evaluated through nursing, medical and legal discourses, with each being informed by different understandings of culture and mental illness. For example, the diagnostic framework of the DSM-5 positions Ruby as a person whose body and mind are disordered, which can be corrected by medication. This separates her from the possibility of maintaining wholeness within her social and cultural context (Wilson, 2008). Nursing is also concerned with her safety, the creation of a safe, protective environment and a trusting relationship.

The delivery of health care happens within a social, cultural and political context. It extends beyond physical and medical diagnoses to beliefs, values, attributes and interpretations from our personal backgrounds. Therapeutically for Cindy and Ruby, these can be held open to different possibilities while working within the constraints of a legislative framework designed to provide for care and protection. Traditionally, Western models of psychiatric and mental health nursing practices have arisen from a biomedical model in which the cultural influences on mental illness have not necessarily been acknowledged. O'Brien and Morrison-Ngatai suggest that 'Western models of mental health care are based on the ideal of disengagement of the self, so that the search for mental health becomes the search for an ideal individual self' (2003, p. 533). Disengagement of self is also disengagement of a cultural self and risks further alienation from Ruby's sense of who she is. So what might this mean? Ruby's ability to maintain control is compromised by a medical diagnosis. At the same time she is trying to make sense and meaning of what is happening to her and her relationships with others. There is a tension between being *locked up* and *not being locked up*. She knows she does not want to be locked up and is unable to say why.

Ruby's desire not be locked up is consistent with the thesis that culturally safe care is defined by the recipient, even though Ruby's behaviour at this time suggests that her ability to make this kind of decision is compromised by her mental state. This creates a paradox for Cindy because a significant component of cultural safety is that 'any action that diminishes, demeans or disempowers the cultural identity and well-being of the individual' is 'not safe care' (Nursing Council of New Zealand, 2011, p. 7). In this scenario not being locked up could be perceived as being safe care for Ruby because it is her stated wish. But Cindy not only has to acknowledge Ruby's wishes, she also has to mediate between providing culturally safe care and working within a legal framework to meet standards for nursing practice. Because of Ruby's compromised situation, her whānau and Cindy are working to maintain her cultural and personal integrity, and well-being in the least restrictive manner.

Culturally specific services such as Kaupapa (policy, philosophy, rules) Māori mental health services may be available for Ruby, her whānau and the in-patient unit team. Their services could include a cultural assessment, karakia (prayer) or whakawhānaungatanga (relationship building). They may be able to help Ruby connect with her sense of wairuatanga (spirituality). A common criticism of mental health services has been the lack of wairuatanga within the assessment and treatment process. Consideration of this factor cannot be underestimated when working with consumers who are Māori and their whānau. As Ruby is known to the service, she may already have a connection with Kaupapa Māori mental health service, or similar, and culturally specific support systems and addictions teams. Cindy can also work with Ruby and her whānau using the recovery approach Blueprint II (2012). A recovery approach is a person-centered approach where service responses focus on the needs of the person rather than the needs of those providing the service. Recovery is based on the premise that services support the engagement of the person and their whānau/family in achieving mental health and well-being thorough a process of recovery. Recovery can be defined as being able to live well in the community with natural supports and within the constraints of living with a mental illness (Blueprint, 2012).

Is Ruby's desire not to be 'locked up' consistent with the definition and standards of culturally safe practice as outlined by the Nursing Council of New Zealand (2011)?

> After leaving the unit, how might Ruby's behaviour put herself and others at risk, and demean, diminish or disempower her cultural identity, and personal and social well-being?
> How would a recovery approach assist Ruby back into attaining a sense of well-being and control?
> How can Cindy use the recovery approach in her relationship with Ruby and her whānau?
> How might a Kaupapa Māori, or similar service, strengthen Ruby's care?
> How might historical factors related to mental illness contribute to Ruby being discriminated against in society?

By highlighting this particular story, we have explored complexity in providing culturally safe practice in mental health nursing. Identifying various discourses or bodies of knowledge through discussion, and cycles of reflecting, re-questioning, redefining and renegotiating events outlined in story, offers some insight into the non-linear nature of culturally safe mental health nursing practice. It also draws attention to the need to attend to the relationship and further understand how power plays out in different situations.

> How might a therapeutic relationship with Ruby look which meets the following multiple needs?
> > Ruby's need for:
> > > safety – cultural, personal, physical, social;

> well-being (freedom from fear and anxiety);
> protection of identity and self-worth;
> freedom from harm.
> Cindy's need to:
>> deliver care in the least restrictive way;
>> be culturally safe;
>> be recovery focused;
>> work with competing discourses of health service delivery.
> If you were taking part in the multidisciplinary team meeting deciding about Ruby's care, how would you contribute? What would you do and say? What would you base your comments on?

Conclusion

Culturally safe care in mental health nursing is complex and multi-layered. It requires the mental health nurse to establish a trusting relationship with clients and understand that relationships are ongoing, with each encounter shaping the next. Nurses act from a conscious, personal and professional understanding of self, with an understanding of the power positions that they hold in their practice. Understanding discourses, and the accompanying values and attitudes operating within particular healthcare settings, enables the nurse to reflect on what is happening in any given situation. An understanding of the socio-political and historical contexts impacting on access to, and appropriate practices within, mental health care can contribute to the enactment of ethical care from a position of self-awareness through reflective practice. Clients are exposed to a number of health and legal discourses, each with their own view of mental illness and the treatment of people with diagnoses of mental illness. With this understanding of differing world views, approaches to care, recovery processes and cultural safety, the nurse is well equipped to develop a therapeutic relationship with the person and their family/whānau. Central to this process is the kaupapa (philosophies) of cultural safety and consumer-driven recovery approaches. That is, that the recipient of care is central to all nursing concerns, actions and achievements, and this care is assessed as being culturally safe by the person receiving the care.

The following table is a representation of how Cindy might frame her practice within the four articles, often referred to as principles, of the Treaty (see Chapter 6 to familiarise yourself with the details). It uses concepts of partnership, protection and participation, as set out in the Royal Commission on Social Policy (1988), to illustrate how Cindy will work with Ruby and her whānau.

TABLE 11.1 *Enacting the principles of partnership protection, participation and tino rangatiratanga (self-determination) in mental health nursing*

ARTICLES OF THE TREATY	MENTAL HEALTH NURSING PRACTICE
Partnership – the principle of Kawanatanga – shared governance	Partnership
The Treaty partnership is between the Crown and tāngata whenua and is representative of all New Zealanders. For Cindy this means improving Ruby's health outcomes in the context of her cultural, personal and mental health needs.	Ruby and her whānau are central to the care that Cindy gives. She works within the parameters of relevant mental health and nursing legislation. She is an active Treaty partner. She takes responsibility for being well informed about the Treaty and understands her own positioning as a mental health nurse, and being from a culture shaped by Western world views and which dominate current health practices. Cindy commits to a process of consultation and negotiation with Ruby and her whānau during all stages and phases of assessment, treatment and recovery. She is able to apply relevant health policies to Ruby's care by accessing specific Māori mental health policies and services. Cindy uses reflexive thinking to monitor the potential for her own internalised prejudice, racism and discriminatory attitudes.
Protection – the principle of Tino Rangatiratanga	Protection
Ruby's sense of self-worth and identity is protected and maintained throughout her hospitalisation and ongoing recovery in her community with her family.	Cindy builds on her previous relationship with Ruby and her whānau, providing an environment that is experienced as culturally, personally and socially safe by Ruby. Ruby is asked about what she does or does not want. Within the parameters of the disinhibiting effects of her present behaviour, she acts as advocate for Ruby and her whānau within the multidisciplinary team. Ruby is given agency/control over her life, as much as she is able, without her coming to harm. Cindy provides an environment which protects Ruby's personal and cultural dignity (Fenton & Te Koutua, 2000).
Participation	Participation
Partnerships cannot be effective unless both partners come from a position of parity and equity. This can be achieved through Ruby, her whānau and Cindy working within a framework of negotiation and consultation.	Cindy understands the role of clients in their power for recovery. Cindy supports Ruby in drawing on her own self-knowledge and expertise in relation to her needs and wants. She works with Ruby and her whānau to help her experience a positive self-image, maintain hope and motivation during this stressful life experience. Cindy will build a therapeutic relationship characterised by consultation, protection and mutual goal-setting with Ruby and her whānau. She will maintain a climate of openness and participation at all levels of care. Cindy creates an environment which reduces the negative impact of stereotyping, racism and discrimination on Ruby's recovery process. Ruby will be provided with information and resources that will help her and her whānau manage her illness, when required, and maintain her dignity, wellness and cultural wholeness when well.
Protection of Māori customs and spiritual freedoms	Protection
This is a verbal agreement between religious leaders and Governor Hobson. It was read before the Treaty meeting prior to the signing of Te Tiriti. It indicates that religious faiths, and Māori customs and religions, shall be protected by him (Governor Hobson, Network Waitangi, 2012, p. 12).	Cindy can work to help continue practices and routines which are important to her as a person and her identity.

References

American Psychiatric Association. (2013). *Diagnostic and statistical manual of mental disorders* (5th edn.). Washington: American Psychiatric Association.

Barker, P. (2001). The Tidal Model: Developing an empowering person-centered approach to recovery within psychiatric mental health nursing. *Journal of Psychiatric Mental Health Nursing, 8*, 233–40.

Blueprint II. (2012). *Improving mental health and wellbeing for all New Zealanders.* Retrieved 18 November 2014 from http://www.hdc.org.nz/media/

Bradley, P. & De Souza, R. (2013). Mental health and illness in Australia and New Zealand. In R.Elde, K. Evans & D. Nizette (eds) *Psychiatric and mental health nursing* (3rd edn.) (pp. 87–108). Sydney: Mosby, Elsevier Australia.

Callaway, B. J. (2002). *Hildegard Peplau: Psychiatric nurse of the century.* New York: Springer.

Carpenter, M. (1980). Asylum nursing before 1914: A chapter in the history of labour. In C. Davies (ed.) *Rewriting nursing history* (pp. 123–46). Surry Hills: Croom-Helm.

Church, O. (1987). The emergence of training programmes for asylum nursing at the turn of the century. In C.Maggs (ed.) *Nursing history: State of the art* (pp. 107—23). North Ryde: Croom-Helm.

Cutliffe, J. & Happell, B. (2009). Psychiatry, mental health nurses, and invisible power: Exploring a perturbed relationship within contemporary mental health care. *International Journal of Advanced Nursing, 18*, 116–25.

Deegan, P. (1992). *Recovery, rehabilitation and the conspiracy of hope.* Lawrence, MA: National Empowerment Centre.

Dinc, L. & Gastmans, C. (2012). Trust and trustworthiness in nursing: An argument based literature review. *Nursing Inquiry, 19*(3), 223–37.doi:10.1111/j.1440-1800.2011.00582.x

Dingwell, R., Rafferty, A. & Webster, C. (1993). *An introduction to the social history of nursing.* London: Routledge.

Durie, M. & Te Kingi, K. (1997). *A framework for measuring Māori mental health outcomes: A report prepared for the Ministry of Health.* Palmerston North: Massey University.

Fenton, L. & Te Koutua, T. W. (2000). *Four Māori Korero about their experience of mental illness.* Wellington: New Zealand Mental Health Commission.

Foucault, M. (1988). *Madness and civilization: A history of insanity in the age of reason,* translated by R. Howard. New York: Vintage Books.

Grant, A. (2003). Freedom and consent. In P. Barker (ed.) *Psychiatric and Mental Health Nursing: The craft of caring.* London: Arnold.

Horsfall, J., Cleary, M. & Hunt, G. (2010). Stigma in mental health: Clients and professionals. *Issues in Mental Health Nursing, 31*, 450–5.

Horsfall, J., Stuhlmiller, C. & Champ, S. (2000). *Interpersonal Nursing for Mental Health*. Sydney: MacLennan and Petty.

Jacob, J., Holmes, D. & Buus, N. (2008). Humanism in forensic psychiatry: The use of the tidal nursing model. *Nursing Inquiry, 15*(3), 224–30.

McEldowney, R. & Connor, M. (2011). Cultural safety as an ethic of care: A praxiological process. *Journal of Transcultural Nursing, 22*(4), 342–9.

Network Waitangi. (2012). *Treaty of Waitangi: Questions and Answers*. Retrieved 21 November 2014 from http://nwo.org.nz/files/QandA.pdf

New Zealand College of Mental Health Nurses. (2012). *Standards of practice for mental health nurses in Aotearoa New Zealand* (3rd edn.). Auckland: New Zealand College of Mental Health Nurses.

New Zealand Government. (2012). Mental Health (Compulsory Assessment and Treatment) Act 1992. Retrieved 21 November 2014 from http://www. health. govt.nz.

Nursing Council of New Zealand. (2005/2011). *Guidelines for cultural safety, the Treaty of Waitangi, and Māori health in nursing education and practice*. Wellington: Nursing Council of New Zealand.

O'Brien, A. & Morrison-Ngatai, E. (2003). Providing culturally safe care. In P. Barker (ed.) *Psychiatric and mental health nursing*. London: Arnold.

O'Hagan, M. (2001). *Recovery competencies for New Zealand mental health workers*. Wellington: Mental Health Commission.

Peplau, H. (1952). *Interpersonal relations in nursing*. New York: Putnam & Sons.

Peplau, H. (1994). Psychiatric mental health nursing: Challenge and change. *Journal of Psychiatric and Mental Health Nursing, 1*, 3–7.

Prebble, K. (2007). Ordinary men and uncommon women: A history of psychiatric nursing in New Zealand public mental hospitals. Unpublished doctoral thesis, University of Auckland, Auckland.

Ramsden, I. (2000). Cultural safety/Kawa Whakaruruhau ten years on: A personal overview. *Nursing Praxis in New Zealand, 15*(1), 4–12.

Ramsden, I. (2002). Cultural safety and nursing education in Aotearoa and Te Waipounamu. Unpublished doctoral thesis, Victoria University of Wellington, Wellington.

Reid, P., Robson, B. & Jones, C. (2000). Disparities in health: Common myths and uncommon truths. *Pacific Health Dialog, 7*(1), 38–47.

Richardson, F. & MacGibbon, L. (2010). Cultural safety: Nurses' accounts of negotiating the order of things. *Women's Studies Journal, 24*(2), 54–65. Retrieved 19 November 2014 from http://wsanz.org.nz/journal/docs/ WSJNZ242RichardsonMacGibbon54-65.pdf

Royal Commission on Social Policy. (1988). *Report of the Royal Commission on Social Policy*. Wellington: Royal Commission on Social Policy.

Rush, B. (2004). Mental health service user involvement in England: Lessons from history. *Journal of Psychiatric and Mental Health Nursing, 11*, 313–18.

Te Pou o Te Whakāro Nui (2009). *Disability Workforce Development*. Auckland: Te Pou.

Travelbee, J. (1971). *Interpersonal aspects of nursing*. Philadelphia: Davis Company.

Watkins, P. (2001). *Mental health nursing: The art of compassionate care*. Oxford: Butterworth-Heinemann.

Wilson, D. (2008). The significance of a culturally appropriate health service for indigenous Māori women. *Contemporary Nurse, 28*, 172–88.

12 Midwifery practice

Katarina Jean Te Huia

Ko te whenua te wai-ūmo nga uri whakatipu.

The ability of the land to sustain human life is likened to the milk from a woman's breast for infants.

Learning objectives

Having studied this chapter, you will be able to:

- consider the historical impact that colonisation has had on the birth culture of Māori;

- apply the principles of cultural safety when caring for Māori women during their antenatal, birth and post-natal experiences;

- consider workforce development issues and cultural safety indicators from the nursing and midwifery professions.

Key terms and concepts

- hapū
- Karakia
- Māori
- Ngā Maia
- Ngā Manukura ō Āpōpō
- pito
- rongoā
- tapu
- tāpuhi
- Turanga Kaupapa
- whakapapa
- whānau
- whare tangata
- whenua

Introduction

This chapter explores some of the traditional cultural concepts around pregnancy and childbirth for Māori. To set the scene, it begins with my journey towards becoming a registered nurse and midwife. An overview of traditional Māori birthing practices and the importance of whakapapa introduces the cultural reality for Māori in terms of whānau. The effect of colonisation is discussed in terms of the introduction of a hospitalised maternity system and the outlawing of traditional home birthing for Māori. Evidence now suggests that the logic, which underpinned the establishment of hospital-based maternity systems, is burdened with inconsistencies that have had a devastating impact on Māori. This chapter therefore focuses on the dominance of medical professionals in maternity care. The client-driven movement for choice, such as woman-centered practices, workforce development issues, and cultural safety, is then addressed in relation to major socio-political issues and influences.

My journey

Practice example

Having completed a diploma in comprehensive nursing in my local area of Hawke's Bay, I pursued a one-year postgraduate diploma in midwifery in Wellington. As a mature student with family commitments, it wasn't an easy decision to leave my loved ones behind on a regular basis and commute out of town for my education. Upon reflection, the journey towards becoming a registered nurse and midwife was the best thing that I ever did, as the benefits have been enormous for myself, my whānau, and, after 20 years, for the community that I have worked in.

At that time (early 1990s), there were no direct-entry midwifery programmes, let alone independent midwives that were Māori, so in many respects I became a 'trailblazer' for Māori women wanting to pursue a career in nursing and midwifery. There is a perception by purists that midwifery should not be 'tainted' by other education or training such as nursing and that to be a midwife one must only be indoctrinated within midwifery. There are definite pros and cons to this argument; suffice it to say there still remain large numbers of registered nurses who manage post-natal wards today in busy District Health Board facilities. There are only four institutes left that offer direct entry midwifery training: AUT, Wintech, Waikato and Otago Polytechnic.

Soon after graduating, I wrote 'Mother and Pepi' as a proposal for the Ministry of Health. It is a clinical assessment programme using a Kaupapa Māori framework to identify vulnerable pregnant Māori women. Together with support from my whānau, I then established a Māori health service. Within this service I established an independent midwifery service for Māori women called 'Choices'. This is a feat I would not recommend to anyone. There was such a great demand from women who wanted to have more choice in their antenatal and post-natal care that the name 'Choices' seemed quite apt for the service. There were also other forces driving me, such as the government's new policy of establishing

Māori health initiatives, Prime Minister Helen Clarke's success in sanctioning changes to maternity services that transformed the midwifery profession into autonomous practitioners for midwives and the devolution of maternity services into the community.

With a Māori-dominated clientele, and five Māori midwives all working together, we were confronted by some of the questions the women put to us. They included:

> 'What should I do with the placenta?' or 'How long can I leave it frozen in the freezer?' and

> 'Is it tapu (forbidden) to go into the urupa (cemetery) when I am hapū? (pregnant)?'

As my education and training in nursing and midwifery was from a Western paradigm, I began my own research beyond the romanticised versions I'd read about. The effects of colonisation had impacted on these women's experiences of pregnancy and childbirth. As a Māori who happened to be a midwife, I felt the weight of Māori women's yearning for cultural knowledge which obviously had not been passed on to me, to them, or to many, if any, of my generation.

Several authors over the years offer accounts of traditional practices related to childbirth (Durie, 1998; Nuku, 2001; Palmer, 2002; Walker, 1990). A key theme they each discuss involves the burial of the whenua back to Papatūānuku, the Earth Mother, soon after the child is born.

This special link with Papatūānuku is evident with the dual meaning given to the term 'whenua'. Whenua can mean 'land' as well as referring to the placenta that feeds the child within the womb. The philosophy here is that through this process, Papatūānuku will continue to feed and sustain the life of all humanity. When buried in ancestral land, the linking of two generations, the past and the present, is reconnecting with 'whakapapa' (genealogy), the ancestors from the past connecting with the offspring of the future. There are variations in this practice from one tribal area to another. Twenty years later, with increasing ethnic diversity, more Māori women are giving birth to babies who are not only from mixed tribal areas, but also from multiracial backgrounds. Many Māori whānau who choose to take their placenta home struggle to complete the process, as they now live in rented accommodation or high rise apartments and, sadly for some, have lost their traditional links with their ancestral lands.

The completed process, therefore, needs to be considered as part of the socio-economic and cultural status of whānau. For the whānau confronted by this dilemma, I ask them to think about a special place for themselves or for their baby. Nowadays, a range of options are considered by whānau such as a seaside reserve, a quiet native bush area, as well as traditional lands.

Traditional Māori birthing

New Zealand's history prior to the arrival of Europeans is constructed from oratory accounts. These accounts were subject to the imagination of the story teller, which could often be influenced as a result of their personal belief. Elsden Best's (1929) beliefs, for example, suggested that Māori were very religious and had a great fear of the supernatural. This was in keeping with his British view of the world where the Christian god was to be feared at all costs and nature was a commodity to be controlled by humankind.

Durie (1998), on the other hand, believed that early Māori were connected to the environment in which they lived. They relied on nature for their survival and developed complex rituals and traditions to keep their own needs, and that of Mother Earth, in balance. They believed that bountiful crops were the results of pleasing the gods and retribution for transgressions against the gods usually resulted in death. Because of their closeness with nature, and their reliance on becoming one with their surroundings, personification of their gods through the naming of mountains, rivers and special places also ensured an account of time and events.

Just as Christian children learned from the Bible that humankind originated from Adam and Eve, Māori children had recounted to them that the beginning of the world stemmed from Ranginui, the Sky Father, and Papatūānuku, the Earth Mother. The world existed in perpetual darkness until the two were forced apart by their children, allowing the light to appear for the first time. Both accounts emphasise the role of women as mothers, nurturers, protectors of the young and propagators for the future. Men are generally perceived as the hunters, warriors and protectors of the family.

Pregnancy and childbirth were considered a normal part of Māori society. Young women observed and contributed to these processes, learning and role modelling each stage of the passages into womanhood. It would have been considered unusual for a female adolescent not to have a clear idea of what to expect with her first pregnancy, given the high level of support and education that was available to her. Her socialisation involved an understanding of her sexuality and the importance of whare tangata or the storehouse of humankind. The reproductive parts of her body were described in this way, since the whare tangata conveyed the importance of women in terms of their capacity to produce future generations.

With this in mind, women were very careful to avoid situations where they may have become infertile. Certain rites and rongoā (remedies) would be taken to either prevent conception or assist fertility (Makereti, 1938). Once a woman became hapū or pregnant, there would be great celebration. This was because the term 'hapū' not only describes pregnancy but also the subtribe of an iwi (tribe). The connection was instantly made between the physical state of infant gestation and the continuation of her people. The celebration would also be for the preservation of whakapapa (genealogy). The concept of whakapapa is still considered by Māori to be the most important concept today as it brings together the connection of kinship groups and a sense of belonging to those groups. A child's whakapapa would always be conveyed to him or her, as this knowledge also carried an expectation that he or she would contribute to the ongoing development and prosperity of the collective.

A pregnant woman was considered tapu (a safety mechanism to protect her and her unborn child) during pregnancy and childbirth. Extra precautions were taken to ensure the spiritual and physical development of the infant was not compromised. These included a restriction on activities by the pregnant woman such as caring for the sick or dying, going into a burial ground or food gathering practices – especially in the sea and waterways, as it was thought that this could bring danger to the unborn child. Also there could be limitations put on eating certain foods, such as fermented corn, so that they benefited from being offered the best food available. This was to ensure the health and well-being for the women during her pregnancy. Procedures for care usually involved a woman's own mother, grandmother, aunt and other female relatives. The use of rongoā (natural medicine) and mirimiri (massage) were important components to prepare the woman's body and check the infant's position.

During the birthing process, a woman would be taken to a special birthing house or whare kohanga (Durie, 1998). It was constructed for this sole purpose and usually destroyed about six weeks post-partum. This ritual confirmed the completion of the tapu process and also facilitated the practical intent of removing any signs that a birth had taken place; a useful strategy if the hapū were required to beat a hasty retreat because of a pending threat. The potential invaders would not possess evidence reflecting the numbers of people in the hapū or the vulnerability of new mothers and babies, thereby limiting the chances of pursuit or capture.

During childbirth, the tāpuhi or midwives used a range of techniques to assist the woman. This included karakia (prayer), waiata (songs), laughter, story telling, rongoā, mirimiri and warm baths. The woman would not lie down during labour, preferring to be in a squatting position. Two vertical posts were constructed for her to brace against and she could also use the knees of the tāpuhi for this purpose. Upon delivery, the baby would have remaining excretions removed by the tāpuhi by taking a deep inward breath over his/her mouth. As the baby took its first breath, a pronouncement to the world could be heard 'Tihei mauri ora!' ('It is the breath of life!'). It is at this moment that the baby is considered to receive a spirit connecting him or her eternally with a tāpuna (ancestor).

The pito (umbilical cord of the baby) would be treated with rongoā to help prevent infection, and the baby would be washed and wrapped. Mirimiri was sometimes performed on the woman until the whenua was delivered soon after. It would then be checked to ensure it was intact. A kete (flax-woven bag) or epu (clay pot) would house the whenua and parapara or meconium until they could be buried at a later date. My aunty Sophie Keefe recounted to me, as a 90-year-old, that when she birthed in her village, she was given a drink made of boiled flax roots, which expelled her placenta and stimulated her milk production. I'm not quite sure if whānau today would engage in these practices as often, as much of this knowledge has been lost.

FOR REFLECTION

> What other cultures do you think shared similar birthing practices to Māori?
> How might you reconcile working with a Māori mother whose baby is from a mixed ethnic heritage?
> The family wants to take their placenta home but are unsure what to do with it. What might you suggest?

Colonisation of Māori birth practices

Following European contact, Māori birthing practices became eroded. New diseases, land confiscations, war, legislation and Christianity had a pervading effect on Māori in all aspects of their life. By 1900, the Māori population was at an all-time low of 42 000, a reduction from 200 000 in 1769 (Pool, 1997).

Diseases such as gonorrhoea and syphilis, and poor living conditions created high levels of sterility for Māori women. For those who gave birth, infant mortality was high, with one in four babies dying during their first year of life (Pool, 1991). With an introduction of alcohol and tobacco, and changes in diet, Māori mothers also suffered from increasing rates of pre-eclampsia, post-partum haemorrhage and maternal death during childbirth (Palmer, 2002). Legislation such as the Midwives Registration Act 1904 and the Tohunga Suppression Act 1907 threatened imprisonment and prevented tāpuhi from continuing to practise traditional birthing within Māori society. The birthing and healing knowledge of tāpuhi and tohunga (experts) were progressively undermined resulting in only minimal information in existence today. A comparison can be drawn with the witch hunts in Europe during the 17th and 18th centuries, when many midwives and women healers were burnt at the stake.

A major turning point for Māori women and the Māori population in general came with reforms introduced by early Māori Members of Parliament – namely,

Āpirana Ngata, Maui Pomare and Te Rangi Hīroa (Peter) Buck. They set about addressing the high mortality rate by focusing on Western methods of hygiene, sanitation, housing and medication (Durie, 1998). However, several obstacles impeded progress in the early 20th century, such as the ethnocentric values of the government and key people such as Truby King, the founder of Plunket. Together they prioritised the rearing of a healthy British population rather than improving the local one (Palmer, 2002).

Maternity care was now the domain of the Education Department's Child Welfare Division under Truby King (Olssen, 1981). Hundreds of independent maternity homes provided childbirth services throughout the country. Seventy-eight per cent of European women were having their babies in hospital, compared with 17 per cent of Māori (Donley, 1986). The 1937 *Commission of Inquiry into Maternity Services in New Zealand* described Māori birthing as involving kneeling or squatting that was not allowed in hospitals, where beds were considered more civilised (Donley, 1986). The racist views that prevailed at that time saw European women reject the idea of sharing hospital services with Māori and chose to travel great distances to avoid this experience (Palmer, 2002).

By the 1940s, the Obstetric Society began to gain power within hospitals and claimed that childbirth was a pathological condition that required medical intervention. This led to the introduction of pain relief and prolonged bed rest within the maternity ward. Hospitalisation for childbirth was not an attractive option for Māori women. Reasons included: the experience of being an unwanted visitor, introduction of indifferent food, the strangeness of hospital staff, prohibition of whānau support, enforcement of the lithotomy position, separation from the baby, giving birth in a place where people die, the burning of the whenua and disrespect for spiritual health (Palmer, 2002).

> Do you think the practices that made Māori reluctant to give birth in hospital are still prevalent? If not, why do you think this is?
> What cultural practices would make our maternity services more acceptable to Māori women today?

The situation today

Throughout the 20th century, medicalised childbirth procedures gained momentum and became routine. By the 1960s, all Māori births took place in a maternity hospital and maternity care was free (Palmer, 2002). Towards the end

184 PART 3: FIELDS OF PRACTICE

of the century, however, women, midwives and pressure groups, such as La Leche League and the New Zealand Home Birth Association, were dissatisfied with the obstetrician-dominated system of care. Their efforts culminated in:

- the establishment of the New Zealand College of Midwives in 1989;
- the reinstatement of direct-entry midwifery programmes (they were abolished in 1957);
- the introduction of the Nurse Amendment Act 1990 (allowing midwives professional status as fully independent providers).

In the past two centuries, Māori have overcome the danger they faced in the 19th century of being a 'dying race' through the efforts of key Māori leaders and health professionals. They have also survived culturally into the 21st century with:

- the advent of Te Kōhanga Reo (Māori language nests) for pre-school children;
- the introduction of the Māori Language Act 1987 which recognised Māori as an official language of New Zealand;
- the passing of the Treaty of Waitangi Acts 1975 and 1985 which acknowledged health as a 'taonga' or treasure for Māori.

The challenge in the 21st century is for Māori women to have their birth practices validated rather than violated. Several approaches, including culturally safe practices, will assist in achieving this goal and result in a healthy population of Māori women, children and whānau. Two of the major approaches follow.

Workforce development

Between 2006 and 2010, the proportion of active Māori midwives was 6–8 per cent of the total active midwifery workforce (Ministry of Health 2011). The number of active Māori midwives increased by 45 or 29 per cent (2006 – 153; 2010 – 198), while the number of all active midwives increased from 2303 to 2639, an increase of 336 or 15 per cent. 'In 2008 the Ministry of Health announced a significant investment into strengthening the Māori workforce. This investment would underpin the government's workforce priority to train more [Māori] nurses and midwives, promote clinical leadership, and increase the size and quality of the frontline clinical workforce. Thus, a national Māori Nursing and Midwifery Workforce Development Programme named Ngā Manukura ō Āpōpō (2014) was established. There is a significant requirement for more

[Māori] clinical leaders in the health and disability sector to help address current and future health service needs. As models of healthcare delivery change, programmes to support both clinical leadership and professional development for Māori nurses and midwives must continue' (Ngā Manukura ō Āpōpō, 2014). In 2014, there are over 3000 registered midwives, with 246 registered Māori midwives. In 1997 the National Body for Māori Midwives, Ngā Maia O Aotearoa, established autonomous regional Ngā Maia affiliates throughout Aotearoa New Zealand. The aim is to support Māori midwifery practice in traditional and Western paradigms, to increase Māori participation in mentoring and supervision for Māori midwifery services, and to participate in discussions and planning into quality Māori maternity care.

Implementation of cultural safety

Over many years health professionals have been engaged and continue to engage in aspects of cultural safety training and as a result are familiar with some aspects of traditional Māori practices. Examples include offering body parts back to Māori after an operation and the return of the placenta to the mother after birth. The option to be cared for by a Māori midwife in most areas of the country is not viable due to the low numbers available. A Māori woman may be asked if she would like a Māori midwife to care for her and sometimes the response is 'Oh, it's OK'. It must not be forgotten that during the period from the signing of the Treaty of Waitangi until the health reforms of the 1990s (King, 2000), Māori were told that they did not have any choice when it came to maternity care. The fact that Māori are offered an informed choice is important. The emphasis on informed choice, however, needs to be genuine and not just a cursory mention of local Māori providers. Partnership is the cornerstone of midwifery practice. The Nursing Council of New Zealand ('the Nursing Council') has some key strategies in place to ensure culturally safe practice. Competencies for registered nurses specifies (but is not limited to):

- **Competency 1.2:** Demonstrates the ability to apply the principles of the Treaty of Waitangi / Te Tiriti o Waitangi to nursing practice.
- **Competency 1.5:** Practices nursing in a manner that the health consumer determines as being culturally safe (Nursing Council of New Zealand, 2007, p. 5).

A set of indicators are provided by the Nursing Council (Nursing Council of New Zealand, 1996) for students to consider as part of their registration requirements as graduates and ongoing professional development. The full version can be found through the Council's website.

The New Zealand College of Midwives' ('the College') philosophy and code of ethics are identified as the foundation of midwifery practice (New Zealand College of Midwives, 2014). Ten practice standards are identified by the College that provide a benchmark for midwives' practice and appropriate usage of midwifery's body of knowledge. Turanga Kaupapa is included as the cultural framework for midwives and adopted by both the Midwifery Council of New Zealand ('the Midwifery Council') and the College. Developed by Nga Maia in 2006, Turanga Kaupapa guidelines are as follows:

- **Whakapapa:** The wahine (woman) and her whānau (family) is acknowledged.
- **Karakia:** The wahine and her whānau may use karakia (prayer).
- **Whanaungatanga**: The wahine and her whānau may involve others in her birthing programme.
- **Te reo Māori:** The wahine and her whānau may speak te reo Māori (Māori language).
- **Mana:** The dignity of the wahine, her whānau, the midwife and others involved is maintained.
- **Hauora:** The physical, spiritual, emotional and mental well-being of the wahine and her whānau is promoted and maintained.
- **Tikanga whenua:** The continuous relationship to land, life and nourishment is maintained; and the knowledge and support of kaumatua and whānau is available.
- **Te whare tangata:** The wahine is acknowledged, protected, nurtured and respected as te whare tangata (the house of people).
- **Mokopuna:** The mokopuna is unique, cared for and inherits the future, a healthy environment, wai u (breastfed) and whānau.
- **Manaakitanga:** The midwife is a key person with a clear role and shares with the wahine and her whānau the goal of a safe, healthy, birthing outcome.

The Midwifery Council's statement on cultural competence for midwives provides a full version of cultural safety indicators that can be downloaded from their website.

FOR REFLECTION

› Examine the competencies and indicators from the Nursing and Midwifery Councils.
› What competencies are similar and what are different?

Conclusion

Traditional Māori birthing practices have been eroded, not only by the medicalisation of childbirth in New Zealand, but also through the attrition of Māori cultural values and the invalidation of tāpuhi and tohunga through legalisation. Two major regulatory authorities such as the Nursing Council and the Midwifery Council have given serious consideration to cultural safety competencies and indicators for engaging with Māori.

Māori need to be encouraged to access the services that best meet their needs, be it a Māori initiative or mainstream services. Within the current environment, Māori whānau are more likely to be urbanised, multiracial and disconnected from their traditional birthing practices. Nurses and midwives are therefore required to improve their engagement with such diverse realities for Māori. The Nursing and Midwifery Councils provide competencies and indicators to support the professions to meet the needs of Māori. A skilled workforce, that is equipped to do so with confidence, can only benefit Māori women and future generations of healthy whānau.

References

Best, E. (1929). *The Whare Kohanga and its lore*. Wellington: Government Printer.

Donley, J. (1986). *Save the Midwife*. Auckland: New Women's Press.

Durie, M. (1998). *Whaiora: Māori health development* (2nd edn.). Auckland: Oxford University Press.

King, A. (2000). *He Korowai Oranga: Māori health strategy*. Wellington: Ministry of Health.

Makereti, M. (1983). *The Old Time Māori*. Auckland: New Women's Press.

Ministry of Health. (2011). *Monitoring the regulated Māori Health Workforce*. Wellington: Ministry of Health.

New Zealand College of Midwives. (2014). *Standards of Practice*. Wellington: New Zealand College of Midwives.

Ngā Manukura ō Āpōpō. (2014). *A National Māori Nursing & Midwifery Workforce Development Programme*. Retrieved 21 November 2014 from http://www.ngamanukura.co.nz/

Nuku, K. (2001). *Māori resource folder: Traditional Māori birth*. Napier: Hawke's Bay District Health Board.

Nursing Council of New Zealand. (1996). *Guidelines for cultural safety, the Treaty of Waitangi, and Māori health in nursing and midwifery education and practice*. Wellington: Nursing Council of New Zealand.

Nursing Council of New Zealand. (2007). *Competencies for registered nurses.* Wellington: Nursing Council of New Zealand.

Olssen, E. (1981). Truby King and the Plunket Society: An analysis of a prescriptive ideology. *New Zealand Journal of History, 15*(1), 3–23.

Palmer, S. (2002). *Hei oranga mo nga wahine hapū (o Hauraki) i roto i te whare ora.* A thesis presented in partial fulfilment of the requirements for the degree of Doctor of Philosophy, University of Waikato, Hamilton.

Pool, I. (1991). *Te Iwi Māori: New Zealand population past, present and projected.* Auckland: Open University Press.

Pool, I. (1997). *The Māori Population of New Zealand 1769–1971.* Auckland: Oxford University Press.

Walker, R. (1990). *Ka Whawhai Tonu Matou: Struggle without end.* Auckland: Penguin.

13

Culturally safe care for ethnically and religiously diverse communities

Ruth De Souza

Learning objectives

Having studied this chapter, you will be able to:

- consider the significance of histories and social relations in shaping knowledge in health;

- examine how liberalism and colonialism are implicated in the Western health system;

- explore how whiteness has shaped nursing education;

- consider how frameworks for addressing inequity in health can reinforce liberal and colonial discourses;

- examine the New Zealand and global context of migration;

- consider indigenous responses to minority cultures: biculturalism and multiculturalism;

- reflect on how cultural safety can be applied to minority populations.

Key terms and concepts

- culture
- cultural safety
- cultural sensitivity
- decolonisation
- indigenous people
- inequality
- liberalism
- migration
- minority populations
- refugees

Introduction

Cultural safety is borne from a specific challenge from indigenous nurses to Western healthcare systems. It is increasingly being developed by scholars and practitioners as a methodological imperative towards universal health care in a culturally diverse world. The extension of cultural safety, outside an indigenous context, reflects two issues: a theoretical concern with the culture of healthcare systems and the pragmatic challenges of competently caring for ethnically and religiously diverse communities.

As discussed throughout this book, the term 'culture' covers an enormous domain and a precise definition is not straightforward. For the Nursing Council of New Zealand ('the Nursing Council') (2009, p. 7), for example, 'culture includes, but is not restricted to, age or generation; gender; sexual orientation; occupation and socioeconomic status; ethnic origin or migrant experience; religious or spiritual belief; and disability'. In an attempt at a precise two-page definition, Gayatri Chakravorty Spivak (2006, p. 359), captures the reflexive orientation required to grasp how the term 'culture' works:

> Every definition or description of culture comes from the cultural assumptions of the investigator. Euro-US academic culture... is so widespread and powerful that it is thought of as transparent and capable of reporting on all cultures. [...] Cultural information should be received proactively, as always open-ended, always susceptible to a changed understanding. [...] Culture is a package of largely unacknowledged assumptions, loosely held by a loosely outlined group of people, mapping negotiations between the sacred and the profane, and the relationship between the sexes.

Spivak's discussion of the sacred and the profane links culture to the more formal institution of religion, which has historically provided the main discourse for discussion of cultural difference. Particularly important for cultural safety is her discussion of Euro-US academic culture, a 'culture of no culture', which has a specific lineage in the sciences of European Protestantism. Through much of the 19th century, for example, compatibility with Christianity was largely assumed and required in scientific and medical knowledge, even as scientists began to remove explicit Christian references from their literature. This historical perspective helps us see how the technoscientific world of the healthcare system, and those of us in secular education, are working in the legacy of white Christian ideals, where the presence of other cultures becomes a 'problem' requiring 'solutions'. Cultural safety, however, attempts to locate the problem where change can be achieved in the healthcare system itself.

The culture of health care

The public health systems in most Western nations were established under a framework of liberal humanism or 'liberalism'. Liberalism is the product of a European culture where the interests of dominant groups are championed at the expense of others, who have not only been ignored and excluded, but enslaved and colonised (Roberts & Sutch, 2004, p. 211). Although liberal humanist arguments have been mobilised to advocate for the equal value of all humans and for equal rights, they have paradoxically also been a mechanism for subordination, as can be seen in the examples of slavery and women not having the vote in many 'free democracies'. What is suppressed in the 'equal treatment' discourse of liberalism are the differences that mark groups out from the people who occupy positions of power and have the authority to legitimate knowledge. There is no level playing field, as qualifying for equality requires that one is assimilated into the worlds of white, Western, bourgeois men who have historically defined what the dominant norms should be, maintaining exclusions despite the promise of inclusion (Bondi, 1993; Roberts & Sutch, 2004).

Western medicine has been viewed as superior for curing disease and restoring health because of its perceived body of objective knowledge that holds 'civilised' Western values such as enlightenment, benevolence and humanitarianism.

This view has come under threat as historians and sociologists have pointed out the political, economic and social imperatives driving medicine and the ends to which it has been put to work (Lewis, 1988). From Christian missionary medicine to biomedicine, the Western health system has participated in the advancement of colonialism and imperialism (Nestel, 2006). Medicine continues to use the language of empire through its claims to modernity and universalism (Anderson, 1998). Western medicine lent moral credibility to the colonial enterprise with discourses of modernity and progress, linking medical knowledge and power with colonial rule (Ejiogu, 2009; Stoler, 1995). It has also used marginalised populations for the 'public' benefit such as in the infamous Tuskegee Study where a control group of

African Americans were falsely told they were receiving syphilis treatment (Gamble, 2008).

While all cultures have ways of caring for others, nursing as a Western profession originated in imperial history and developed during the industrialisation of medicine, maintaining many colonial features (Gilbert, 2003). Florence Nightingale, who developed sanitary reforms and administrative skills during Britain's imperial campaign in the Crimea, is known as the originator of modern nursing in the European tradition. Nightingale made practical contributions to the imperial enterprise, through the founding of the Nightingale Training School for Nurses in 1860 that then became the model for similar establishments throughout the British Empire (Fahy, 2007).

Browne (2001) has identified four ways in which liberal ideology shapes nursing: the individualistic focus of nursing science; nurses' view of society as essentially egalitarian; a preference for politically neutral knowledge development; and the economy of knowledge development in nursing (p. 123). She suggests that, in combination, they individualise the responsibility for health access and maintenance, while rendering invisible the larger social conditions that contribute to individuals' ability to take this responsibility. The ideology of egalitarianism rests on the notion that all individuals are on a 'level playing field' with equal access to health services and equal resources to achieve health. Within this framework, if you are unhealthy or have difficulty accessing health care, it is your own fault or an individual deficit (2001). Browne contends that the advent of strategies such as multiculturalism, diversity and indigenous rights can lull us into believing that systemic inequities are being rectified. However, the continuing persistence of inequality has prompted a continuing search for new paradigms that consider the historical, cultural, social and economical forces that shape knowledge development (Browne, 2001; Jowett & O'Toole, 2006).

Allen (2006, p. 66) also notes the 'white supremacy' of nursing education, suggesting that its curricular machine with predetermined outcomes and mechanisms is based on an assimilationist agenda, where adding 'other' people into the mainstream creates a multicultural environment. This addition reinforces rather than displaces whiteness from the centre of structures and processes of educational or clinical institutions. Therefore multiculturalism must encompass 'some vision of political negotiation theorized within a historical understanding of cultural dominance if progress is to occur' (p. 67). Allen proposes a critical multiculturalism, where representations of difference from multiple, heterogeneous perspectives are developed, and democratic conversations with multiple voices are undertaken, so that other cultural perspectives can be legitimated and previously suppressed histories made explicit (2006).

What specific strategies can be employed towards culturally safe care?

Joan Scott suggests that the ideology of being a 'nice' person as sufficient care can be depoliticising, shifting emphasis from the social and historical to the personal or cultural:

> There is nothing wrong, on the face of it, with teaching individuals about how to behave decently in relation to others and about how to empathize with each other's pain. The problem is that difficult analyses of how history and social standing, privilege, and subordination are involved in personal behavior entirely drop out. (1992, p. 9)

Responses for clinicians typically feature 'cultural sensitivity', mobilising culturalist discourses to de-emphasise limitations in liberal commitments to equity and universal access to health care. Culturalist discourses are 'the complex practices and ideologies that use popularized, stereotyped representations of culture, often conflated with ethnicity, as the primary analytical lens for understanding presumed differences about various groups of people' (McConaghy, 1997, cited in Browne & Varcoe, 2006, p. 158). The political neutralising of a critical anti-racist agenda in care is another effect of culturally sensitive frameworks in nursing (Culley, 2006).

Cultural sensitivity frameworks (or transculturalism) have reinforced liberal and colonial discourses. Such discourses have individualising and culturalising impacts which maintain the status quo, and produce, and reproduce, inequality. In such a framework, the remedy for the problem of caring across difference is integration. The health professional becomes more sensitive or knowledgeable about other cultures and the person from a racialised group becomes more like the dominant culture (Reed, 2003). Integration assumes an already formed national culture with universal values possessed by the dominant culture into which newcomers must be incorporated. However, the apparent promise of inclusion preserves a racial hierarchy rather than dissolves it (Razack, 2004) and attenuates demands for structural change.

Cultural awareness and sensitivity training can be useful ways to stimulate self-reflection and a historical sensibility if there isn't an institutional response and the responsibilities for institutional racism remain individualised. Cultural safety demands self-reflexivity (unlike the other two approaches), where the gaze is directed at the self, to account for one's own role as a culture bearer rather than displacing culture onto the 'other' as different (Ramsden, 1997; 2000; 2002). Cultural safety does not aim to describe the practices of other ethnic groups because such a strategy can lead to a checklist mentality that essentialises group members (Nursing Council of New Zealand, 2002). Furthermore, a nurse having knowledge of a client's culture could be regarded as disempowering for a client who is disenfranchised from his or her own culture, and could be seen as the continuation of a colonising process that is both demeaning and disempowering (Ramsden, 2002), or inappropriate (Allen, 1999). Culturally safe nurses focus on self-understanding, and recognising the attitudes and values nurses bring to their practice. A key tenet is that 'a nurse or midwife who can understand his or her own culture and the theory of power relations can be culturally safe in any context' (Nursing Council of New Zealand, 2002, p. 8). The progression towards culturally safe practice occurs in three steps:

1 cultural awareness, which involves understanding that there is difference;
2 cultural sensitivity, where difference is legitimated, leading to self-exploration;
3 cultural safety, the outcome of nursing and midwifery education where recipients of care define safe service (Ramsden, 2002).

When helping doesn't help

Practice example

Many years ago, when I moved from working in community mental health to a maternity ward, I was instructed to give a Chinese woman, who'd recently given birth, an ice pack for her perineum as this was the policy on the post-natal ward I worked on. She refused, saying that she needed to keep warm. A couple of years after this incident, when I was working as a member of the maternal mental health team, I went to visit a Sri Lankan mother of twins. When I advised her of the service that I was able to provide, involving medications and talk therapies, she announced 'I don't need any of that. I need someone to give me practical help – to wash nappies, to help with the housework and to cook.'

Both these examples led me to think deeply about how helping sometimes doesn't help, especially if the help that's on offer isn't what someone needs. Yet how can we resolve these differences about what is seen as helpful when the help on offer is geared toward the needs and values of the dominant culture? That question has remained with me throughout my career. We can't assume that routine practice or what we think is helpful will necessarily be helpful to someone operating from a different set of values and beliefs. This makes it important to have a conversation with the person and ensure that our care is always client-centred.

Minority populations and migration

In 2013, one in four New Zealanders was born overseas with Asia being the most common region of birth. Of those born overseas, the top three countries of birth were England, China and India. This diversity of place of birth has been accompanied by linguistic and religious diversity. The top four languages spoken in New Zealand were English, Māori, Samoan and Hindi. Although the European ethnic group was the largest, almost three quarters of the population identified with one or more European ethnicity (Statistics New Zealand, 2013). A percentage breakdown of the population in 2013 was as follows:

- Māori: 14.9 per cent;
- Asian: 11.8 per cent;
- Pacific: 7.4 per cent;
- Middle Eastern/Latin American/African: 1.2 per cent (Statistics New Zealand, 2013).

Migration can be motivated by 'pull' factors, where migrants are drawn to a new country for the opportunities that are available or due to 'push' factors, when they leave a place due to a range of issues in their home nation.

Migrants are people who were born in one country and then move to another under an immigration programme. In New Zealand this consists of several categories[1]:

- Skilled migrant – relates to attracting migrants with qualifications and skills;
- Business – relates to attracting money or business expertise and enabling experienced business people to create business opportunities in New Zealand;
- Family sponsored – New Zealand citizens or permanent residents can sponsor family members to enter the country;
- Humanitarian – this includes refugees and allows for family members to be granted residence if there are serious humanitarian concerns.

Different histories and patterns of migration have shaped contemporary Aotearoa New Zealand. Polynesian groups first settled in about AD 1300. Europeans began arriving after 1769, with organised settlement occurring from 1840. Waves of kin migration through favourable policies soon resulted in a dominance of Pākehā, with Māori becoming outnumbered by settlers. The

---

[1] There are also categories that acknowledge the longstanding relationships with our Pacific neighbours: the Samoan Quota and the Pacific Access.

Treaty of Waitangi established a formal relationship between Māori and the British Crown; however, visibly different migrants, such as Indians, Chinese and Samoans, became 'others' because they were neither Māori nor Pākehā, and because of differences in religion or culture. Restrictive Acts of Parliament ensued between 1870 and 1899 that prevented Chinese from owning land, for example. The Acts were only repealed when new sources of labour were required.

Global capitalism drives migration flows and governmental policies have always supported industries to obtain 'new' workers. In New Zealand, for example, the 1970s saw the arrival of many Pacific Island migrants as part of a labour shortage in the manufacturing sector. In the neo-liberal era, which features high unemployment in wealthier nations, foreign direct investment has become a primary goal of the state, the sought after migrants are high net worth individuals. Countries now compete for such migrants, searching beyond traditional source countries for newcomers (for example in the case of New Zealand, migrants traditionally came from the United Kingdom and mainland Europe but now also come from Asia). Where homogeneity was once a migration filter, the competition for migrants globally has required migrants who can be assimilated (Camiscioli, 2001). Additionally, the presence of war and lack of access to human rights have resulted in forced migration, noticeable in the growing number of refugees.

In 2013, there were estimated to be 51.2 million refugees, asylum seekers and displaced people worldwide in need of protection and help (United Nations Refugee Agency, 2013 (UNHCR)). More than 80 per cent are women and children.

There are two ways in which refugees are able to remain in New Zealand. The first is the 'quota category', which in New Zealand is presently 750 people per year, a figure that has remained unchanged since 1987. Quota refugees receive a structured resettlement programme of six weeks duration. People are recommended by the UNHCR to Immigration New Zealand for selection. The refugees who apply for resettlement in New Zealand must meet the definition of a refugee. The second resettlement category includes convention refugees or asylum seekers who have numbered approximately 100 per year in recent years compared to approximately 350 prior to increased surveillance following 9/11. However, asylum seekers have minimal access to support services (Global Detention Project, 2014).

The word 'convention' refers to the United Nations' 1951 *Convention Relating to the Status of Refugees* – a key legal document outlining the rights of refugees and the legal obligations of signatory states. Article 1 (2) of the United Nations' 1967 *Protocol Relating to the Status of Refugees* modifies Article 1 A (2) of the 1951 Convention to define a 'refugee' as a person who:

> owing to a well-founded fear of being persecuted for reasons of race, religion, nationality, membership of a particular social group or political opinion, is outside the country of his nationality and is unable or, owing to such a fear, is unwilling to avail himself of the protection of that country; or who, not having a nationality and being outside the country of his former habitual residence, is unable or, owing to such fear, is unwilling to return to it.

This definition only refers to people who have fled their country of origin and then sought sanctuary in a second country for protection.

New Zealand ranks 88th in the world for hosting refugees per capita. This works out to one refugee per year for every 6000 New Zealanders. In comparison, Australia takes in one refugee for every 1175 Australians (Stephens, 2014).

Decolonisation

Decolonisation is an additional driver of the need for culturally responsive care and the cultural safety movement. After World War II, the *Charter of the United Nations* (see Article 73) coincided with a withdrawal of European powers from former colonies. For those nations, the legacy colonial infrastructure had to adapt to local cultural conditions, while many from the former colonies would continue their movement to Europe. The process of decolonisation was not solely at the nation's state level, however, but also became important for indigenous people in white settler societies, where colonial governments gained independence, as they struggled for the acknowledgement of their human rights.

Inequalities in health

Pacific peoples, Asian peoples and Middle Eastern, Latin American and African (MELAA) communities in white settler societies receive a different quality of care, as seen by disparities between the health of these groups and Pākehā. In New Zealand, Pacific people are the least likely of any ethnic group to access primary care. Their rates of avoidable deaths, hospitalisations and ambulatory-sensitive hospitalisations are higher than in non-Pacific populations. Asian communities have historically been the main targets of exclusionary immigration legislation.

In Australia and New Zealand they continue to receive unwelcome media and political attention, despite making up 11.8 per cent of the population. One issue in the provision of public health for these groups is a lack of available data. This reflects migration's involvement in the shift from a population management approach by the state to a neoliberal capitalist model.

Innovative health models have been developed to address Pacific health inequalities such as the Fonofale model as well as 'for and by Pacific' services. A growing body of research is being developed to guide the health needs of Asian people and MELAA communities.

What narratives (dominant, migrant, indigenous) apply to your own citizenship in your nation?

Indigenous responses to minority cultures: mana whenua and manuhiri

While multiculturalism has been developed in European nation states as a tool to manage diverse groups, this has also caused tension in indigenous settings where treaty-based negotiations of sovereignty with colonial powers are displaced into discourses of culture. The result has been that for many indigenous people, discussions of multiculturalism are correctly seen as attempts to dilute the significance of competing claims to self-determination. Biculturalism (the recognition of indigenous culture's specific role in the nation) is then opposed to multiculturalism as a pluralist form of cultural management.

However, a number of critical educators have explained that bicultural and multicultural discourses need not be opposed. Under a framework of Tangata Tiriti, for example, the diversity of new arrivals to Aotearoa can be acknowledged, even as the underlying structure of the nation state is assumed. Yet all indigenous groups have their own forms of managing cultural differences in questions of political authority and cultural protocol. Within Māori, for example, a discourse of tangata whenua (hosts) and manuhiri (visitors) establishes expectations of intercultural engagement, noting that even within 'Māori culture' there are debates and contests over tikanga (values) and kawa (protocol) that must be negotiated. The concept of 'mana whenua' (authority deriving from the land) provides the grounding principle that facilitates the arrival of visitors to a new land, one that is often more hospitable than European forms of cultural management.

Conclusion

Given the growing evidence of health inequalities among the groups outlined earlier in this chapter, an investigation of the care of minority populations requires an examination of how clinical encounters reflect broader coagulations of power. To date, the behaviours, dispositions and cultures of migrants have received greater scholarly attention than the institutional and structural contingencies that shape their lives. International evidence shows that racialised patients are often viewed negatively and receive care from health professionals that ignores or denigrates their culturally specific needs. Issues at stake include:

- different conceptions of what constitutes caring;
- language and communication problems;
- poor access to appropriate information;
- barriers to accessing care;
- cultural competence;
- tensions between models of care;
- tensions between professional intervention and family and community involvement (Bowes & Domokos, 1998; Davies & Bath, 2001; Wikberg & Bondas, 2010).

Health practitioners construct ethnic users of health services negatively and withhold recognition of their needs, seeing cultural needs as belonging to the private sphere, rather than a public health system, providing universal services (Davies & Papadopoulos, 2006).

The implementation of cultural safety in a multicultural context requires that nurses explore the histories and social relations that shape our knowledge and have discriminatory effects. The knowledges that underpin the practices of nurses and midwives are neither neutral nor innocent; instead they reflect specific histories and cultural values and are imbued with power. Rather than an innocent decontextualised meeting between clinician and other, the ethnically different body reflects a contested realm historically inscribed with hierarchical social relations. The decolonising power of feminism can be activated if consideration is given to how maternity and motherhood in the West have been constituted through relationships with colonialism, capitalism and patriarchy (Lentin 2004).

Ultimately, the nursing profession must become more political than its 'supportive' role to biomedicine has traditionally entailed. In order to provide ongoing culturally appropriate care, nursing must address its conservative allegiances to patriarchal and bureaucratic practices, which have prevented it from engaging in its own transformation (Walker & Holmes, 2008). Nursing's liberal repertoire should open towards an acknowledgement of the uncertain, contradictory and highly politicised nature of its knowledge production and consider' new methodological resources, new metaphors and practical strategies' (Burman 2006, p. 17). Cultural safety provides an opportunity to destabilise taken-for-granted constructions and practices, allowing truly universal care to be pursued in a globalising and complex world.

FOR
REFLECTION

> What values are evident in the healthcare institutions you encounter (for example, self-responsibility)?
> To what extent do the dominant values of the institutions align or misalign with your own?
> Have you been involved in a caring situation where your actions may have been received differently than you expected?
> Do you have family connections in other parts of the world? If so, how did your family come to be in different places?
> What might be some 'push' factors that lead people to leave their home country?
> What might be some 'pull' factors that lead people to move to a particular country?
> Do you think the refugee quota should be increased?
> What initiatives could you start in your own place of work or study towards culturally safe care?

Although cultural safety emerges from indigenous critiques of the colonial health system, it is an important tool for all those using human rights and social justice approaches to transform the health system. Its key feature is the identification of the practitioner and institution as a culture-bearing entity, removing the burden of culture from the patient and placing the encounter of care as an opportunity for transformation in power relations. It thus opens the potential for the increasing complexity of cultural flows in the health system to be seen as a springboard for rethinking default understandings of culture and power, shifting nurses from relatively powerless biomedical handmaidens to strategically positioned advocates for universal care. This commitment to the patient as a site of cultural encounter rather than a cultural problem undoubtedly causes challenges for practitioners and managers within a monocultural health system which focuses on efficiency and cost-reduction. However, if the essence of nursing lies with patient advocacy, alliances with patient's cultural needs and committing to the never-achieved process of cultural discovery will only strengthen the capability of practitioners and the healthcare profession as a whole.

References

Allen, D. G. (1999). Knowledge, politics, culture and gender: A discourse perspective. *Canadian Journal of Nursing Research, 30*(4), 277–34.

Allen, D. G. (2006). Whiteness and difference in nursing. *Nursing Philosophy, 7*(2), 65–78.

Anderson, W. (1998). Where is the postcolonial history of medicine? *Bulletin of the History of Medicine, 72*, 522–30.

Bondi, L. (1993). Locating identity politics. In M. Keith & S. Pile (eds.) *Place and the politics of identity* (pp. 84–101). London; New York: Routledge.

Bowes, A. M. & Domokos, T. M. (1998). Health visitors work in a multi-ethnic society: A qualitative study of social exclusion. *Journal of Social Policy, 27*(4), 489–506.

Browne, A. J. (2001). The influence of liberal political ideology on nursing science. *Nursing Inquiry, 8*(2), 118–29.

Browne, A. J. & Varcoe, C. (2006). Critical cultural perspectives and health care involving Aboriginal peoples. *Contemporary Nurse, 22*(2), 155–67.

Burman, E. (2006). (How) can critical psychology help female antiracist work? *Critical Psychology*, (8), 9–34.

Camiscioli, E. (2001). Producing citizens, reproducing the "French race": Immigration, demography, and pronatalism in early twentieth-century France. *Gender and History, 13*(3), 593–621.

Culley, L. (2006). Transcending transculturalism? Race, ethnicity and health-care. *Nursing Inquiry, 13*(2), 144–53.

Davies, M. M. & Bath, P. A. (2001). The maternity information concerns of Somali women in the United Kingdom. *Journal of Advanced Nursing, 36*(2), 237–45. doi:10.1046/j.1365-2648.2001.01964.x

Davies, M. M. & Papadopoulos, I. (2006). Notions of motherhood and the maternity needs of Arab Muslim women. In I. Papadopoulos (ed.) *Transcultural health and social care: The development of culturally competent practitioners* (pp. 145–63). London: Elsevier.

Ejiogu, N. (2009). "A clinic for the world": Race, biomedical citizenship, and gendered national subject formation in Canada. Unpublished Masters thesis, University of Toronto, Toronto.

Fahy, K. (2007). An Australian history of the subordination of midwifery. *Women and Birth, 20*(1), 25–9.

Gamble, V. (2008) [2003]. The enduring legacy of Tuskegee Syphilis Study, *LeNoir – NMA Pediatric Lecture Series*. Retrieved 6 November 2010 from http://www.youtube.com/watch?v=CJa4Qd-FB70

Gilbert, H. (2003). Great adventures in nursing: Colonial discourse and health care delivery in Canada's north. *Jouvert: A Journal of Postcolonial Studies, 7*(2)

(Winter/Spring 2003). Retrieved 1 September 2014 from http://english.chass. ncsu.edu/jouvert/v7i2/gilber.htm

Global Detention Project. (2014). New Zealand detention profile. Retrieved 1 September 2014 from http://www.globaldetentionproject.org/countries/asia-pacific/new-zealand/introduction.html

Jowett, M. & O'Toole, G. (2006). Focusing researchers' minds: Contrasting experiences of using focus groups in feminist qualitative research. *Qualitative Research*, 6(4), 453–72.

Lentin, R. (2004). Strangers and strollers: Feminist notes on researching migrant m/others. *Women's Studies International Forum*, 27(4), 301–14.

Lewis, M. (1988). The 'health of the race' and infant health in New South Wales: Perspectives on medicine and empire. In R. M. MacLeod & M. J. Lewis (eds.) *Disease, medicine, and empire: Perspectives on Western medicine and the experience of European expansion* (pp. 301–15). London: Routledge.

Nestel, S. (2006). *Obstructed labour: Race and gender in the re-emergence of midwifery.* Vancouver: UBC Press.

New Zealand Nursing Council. (2009). *Guidelines for cultural safety, the Treaty of Waitangi and Māori health in nursing education and practice.* Wellington: New Zealand Nursing Council.

Nursing Council of New Zealand. (2002). *Guidelines for cultural safety, the Treaty of Waitangi and Māori health in nursing and midwifery education and practice* (p. 24). Wellington: Nursing Council of New Zealand.

Ramsden, I. (1997). Cultural safety: Implementing the concept – the social force of nursing and midwifery. In P. T. Whaiti, M. McCarthy, & A. Durie (eds.) *Mai i rangiatea* (pp. 113–25). Auckland: Auckland University Press and Bridget Williams Books.

Ramsden, I. (2000). Cultural safety/kawa whakaruruhau ten years on: A personal overview. *Nursing Praxis in New Zealand, 15*(1), 4–12.

Ramsden, I. (2002). Cultural Safety and Nursing Education in Aotearoa and Te Waipounamu. Unpublished doctoral thesis, Victoria University, Wellington.

Razack, S. (2004). Imperilled Muslim women, dangerous Muslim men and civilised Europeans: Legal and social responses to forced marriages. *Feminist Legal Studies, 12*(2), 129–74.

Reed, K. (2003). *Worlds of health: Exploring the health choices of British Asian mothers* (pp. xii, 191). Westport; London: Praeger.

Roberts, P. & Sutch, P. (2004). *An introduction to political thought: Key concepts and thinkers.* New York: New York University Press.

Scott, J. W. (1992). Multiculturalism and the politics of identity. *October, 61,* 12–19.

Spivak, G. C. (2006). Culture alive. *Theory, Culture & Society, 23*(2–3), 359–60. doi:10.1177/026327640602300264

Statistics New Zealand. (2013). *Census quickstats about national highlights.* Retrieved 1 September 2014 from http://www.stats.govt.nz/Census/2013-census/profile-and-summary-reports/quickstats-about-national-highlights.aspx

Stephens, M. (2014). Miserly refugee intake shows New Zealand has to do more. *Dominion Post.* Retrieved 1 September 2014 from http://www.doingourbit. co.nz/p/the-issue.html

Stoler, A. L. (1995). *Race and the education of desire: Foucault's history of sexuality and the colonial order of things* (pp. xiv, 237). Durham: Duke University Press.

United Nations General Assembly. (1951). *Convention relating to the status of refugees, 28 July 1951.* Retrieved 1 September 2014 from http://www.refworld.org/ docid/3be01b964.html

United Nations General Assembly. (1967). *Protocol relating to the status of refugees, 31 January 1967.* Retrieved 1 September 2014 from http://www.refworld.org/ docid/3ae6b3ae4.html

United Nations Refugee Agency (2013). *Global forced displacement tops 50 million for first time since World War II.* Retrieved 1 September 2014 from http://www.unhcr. org/53a155bc6.html

Walker, K. & Holmes, C. (2008). The 'order of things': Tracing a history of the present through a re-reading of the past in nursing education. *Contemporary Nurse, 30*(2), 106–18.

Wikberg, A. & Bondas, T. (2010). A patient perspective in research on intercultural caring in maternity care: A meta-ethnography. *International Journal of Qualitative Studies on Health and Well-Being, 5*(1). doi:10.3402/qhw.v5i1.4648

14 Working with the aged

LESSONS FROM RESIDENTIAL CARE

Liz Kiata and Ngaire Kerse

Learning objectives

Having studied this chapter, you will be able to:

- explore culturally related differences in attitudes and beliefs about being old;

- examine the potential impact of culturally related differences on care practices, especially:
  › views and expectations about being older;
  › communication and language;
  › racism;
  › power relationships.

Key terms and concepts

- ageist attitudes

- belief systems

- ethnic groups

- intercultural care

- reciprocal relationship

- residential care

Introduction

Frail older residents living in one long-term care facility and the nurses, caregivers and healthcare assistants caring for them, took part in a field study (Kiata & Kerse, 2004). In the facility, which was located in a large New Zealand city, most of the health professionals were of Pacific Island descent and the majority of residents were European (Pākehā). The purpose of the study was to explore how Pacific Island caregivers and Pākehā care recipients in the facility negotiated their way through the giving and receiving of care.

Intercultural issues that arose are examined and used in this chapter as illustrative examples.

Caregivers were sanctioned by management to participate in the research and encouraged by reassurances of confidentiality. Caregivers were interviewed by two researchers – one young man of Pacific origin, the other a middle-aged Pākehā woman. The frailty of the residents meant that they tired quickly, so shorter interviews were conducted. Residents were quick to become teary during interviews. This may have been part of certain illnesses, such as stroke, or these emotional outbursts may also have been due to the interest shown when asked to share their stories. Certainly, the majority stated that the 'nurses' were 'always so busy' (Miss E, 90s),[1] and how they were reluctant to bother them. Participant observation was added to interview data, and information and understanding through thematic analysis. Conducting this research gave insight into the everyday lives of those who live and work in residential care.

The multiple cultural aspects of care (given and received) that are voiced in this chapter are 'acted on and given meaning' through a number of viewpoints (Denzin, 1994, p. 509). These points of view are based on, but not exclusive to, cultural, ethnic and gender perspectives. We encourage you to think about the material presented and interpret the findings through a filter made up from their own perspectives and life experiences. It is important to note that, although there may be several interpretations of similar situations and reportings, no one view is likely to be considered 'strictly' correct. We hope that you will reflect on this chapter and use these reflections to inform your own interactions with culturally diverse people encountered throughout, not only in your employment setting, but also your everyday lives.

The Auckland Ethics Committee approved the study. A major report, containing an expanded version of the information in this chapter, was circulated to management and staff in the home for discussion. All staff and residents are referred to by pseudonyms in publications and staff generally agreed that they could not identify themselves or others from comments stated in the report.

While the field study concentrated on ethnic groups, culturally based issues can be considered relevant to other cultural groups. It would be inappropriate to directly extrapolate these views to other minority groups and unrealistic to cover all ethnicities in one chapter. We encourage you to use your own

---

[1] Pseudonyms are used when referring to participants.

experiences, knowledge and information from relevant community groups and the literature to inform learning about intercultural care.

For clarity in this chapter, all staff employed at the facility, irrespective of qualifications or position held in the workplace, will be termed 'health carers' and the elders who live at there will be named 'residents'.

Residential care

> Care … is not a marginal activity of life but one of the central procedures of human existence. Care is not confined to the family or personal relationships but is also situated in formalised social and political institutions in our society. (Sevenhuijsen, 1998, p. 137).

Along with other developed countries including Australia, the United Kingdom and the United States, New Zealand is following a global trend towards an ever-growing aging population (Organisation for Economic Cooperation and Development, 1996). On an international level, this means that quality in residential care will be of increasing interest to health professionals, consumers, health funders and researchers over the next decades – and there is room for improvement.

Older people living in residential aged care have become older, frailer and more dependent (Boyd et al., 2009). Within this aged care setting, the giving of care represents a complex mix of vulnerable frail, older care recipients, underpaid and overworked staff, and an organisational setting that potentially impacts on care. With an increasing ethnically diverse population, a workforce consisting of health professionals from diverse cultural and ethnic backgrounds meets the daily needs of these residents.

What is known about living and working in residential care is mainly based on nursing homes through ethnographic studies conducted in the United States. Physical and psychological abuse 'we know, is distressingly common' (Foner, 1995, p. 39) in the United States, and in the United Kingdom 'old folks homes' have been termed 'workhouses' in past times and viewed negatively (Wilson, 2000, cited in Kiata & Kerse, 2004).

Residential care for older New Zealanders emerged in the late 1960s, care and mis-care (sic) of the aged being described in the literature (Department of Health, 1988; North Shore Old People's Welfare Council, 1969). More recent New Zealand-based research (Peri et al., 2008; Wilkinson et al., 2012), along with policy developments, emphasise the maintenance of health and independence in residential care settings, and the principle of respect and positive caring environ-ments underpin policy direction (for example, Ministry of Health, 2013).

The giving and receiving of care is complex. Key components of successful caregiving involve:

- sensitivity;
- acting in the best interest of others;
- engaging in the process of a reciprocal relationship between the giver and receiver of care (Tarlow, 1996).

> How is the process of caring for very frail, older people different from caring for people recovering from an acute illness in hospital?

> How do you think carers supporting older people living in long-term residential care manage the day-to-day pressures of caring for people who are very frail?

FOR REFLECTION

In the residential care setting, several levels of staff are involved in the organisa-tion of care delivery. These include managerial staff, registered nurses, health-care assistants, as well as support staff, such as cooks and cleaners. Interac-tions at all levels are affected by power relationships: employer to employee; nurse to healthcare assistant; healthcare assistant to frail, older person. At all levels, cultural and ethnic diversity add to the complexity of these relation-ships. Dynamics of ethnicity, culture and gender influence exacerbate divi-sions between groups (Foner, 1995). Healthcare assistants may feel quite dis-empowered as low wages keep them at the margins of subsistence income and underline the workforce's status. More often than not, this workforce is female (Diamond, 1992, cited in Kiata & Kerse, 2004). As the residents can be con-sidered to be increasingly vulnerable, they become continuously dependent on health carers for their everyday activities.

Keeping in mind this complex context, culturally related beliefs of the health carers and the residents will now be discussed.

Intercultural care

Ethnically based cultural beliefs about ageing can influence health and must be taken into consideration (Gallant, Sptize & Grove, 2010). Cultural groups have differing views about being old, ageing, how to best care for older people and who should provide care. Substantial numbers of those currently caring for older peo-ple in residential care in New Zealand and overseas are of non-European descent while the residents they care for are from all ethnicities but tend to be mainly

Pākehā (Kiata & Kerse, 2004). While 'reasons for this are not entirely clear, a mix of culturally related attitudes to ageing, financial barriers, and the perception that ethnic minority elders are not safe in residential care culminate to mean that ethnic minority residents are under-represented in residential care' in New Zealand (Kiata & Kerse, 2004, p. 315). Factors such as low remuneration and rigid hierarchy contribute to the workforce consisting mainly of people from ethnic minority groups (Kiata & Kerse, 2004).

Culturally and ethnically related belief systems

Culturally and ethnically related views encountered during the field study are summarised into views about ageing, food, physical demands of care, status, racism and communication. The relevance of these issues to caregiving is discussed.

Views about being older

Aging happens in a cultural context (Fry, 2000, p. 751). For Pacific Islanders , caregiving plays an important and relevant role within their own culture. Caregiving work may be seen as an 'extension of previous experiences with looking after the emotional and physical needs of infirm family members' (Kiata & Kerse, 2004, p. 321). During the field study, Pacific Island healthcare assistants believed that these traits distinguished them from Pākehā who, in the health carers' eyes, tended to 'leave the caring of "their" elders to others... in institutionalized settings' (Carer P, cited in Kiata & Kerse, 2004, p. 322). Pacific Island health carers were said to be 'better than others [ethnicities] because they respect their elders' (Carer I, cited in Kiata & Kerse, 2004, p. 321). Furthermore, the caring role and patient nature of Pacific Islanders who look after their elders was believed to assist them in the workplace.

A common theme running through the narratives of health carers was perceived cultural differences in aged care practices. They discussed the investment that Pacific Islanders have in caring for their children and were of the belief that this care will be returned in kind by their children who will care for them in their old age (Kiata & Kerse, 2004).

> Contrary to this philosophy, [they reported that] Pākehā people rely on monetary investments to ensure care for their older years. For elderly

people, there comes a time when an independent lifestyle is no longer possible, and cashing in their investments becomes necessary. For Pākehā, this means having to pay for long-term care (usually) in a residential setting away from their homes, and strangers provide the care required. For Pacific Islander elders, however, the earlier investment in their young people means that the children, now grown, will care for them as elders within a familial context. (Kiata & Kerse, 2004, p. 318)

The main point of difference between views about elders may lie in the degree of 'mutual trust and respect between the elderly and the young' (Kiata & Kerse, 2004, p. 318) as illustrated in Figure 14.1. Health carers noted several distinctions. The concept of 'active agency' was one of these distinctions. For instance, from the researchers' experiences with Samoan etiquette, 'the relationship between the carer (usually a young person) and the elderly is marked by fa'aaloalo (respect) and alofa (love), and is mutually understood as such' (Kiata & Kerse, 2004, p. 319). Old age for Pacific Islanders means a form of submission and little active agency regarding the type of care received.

Basic necessities such as food and physical care are given to the elderly at the carer's discretion. However, the older person and the caregiver understand that submitting to the role of 'cared for' does not necessarily mean loss of empowerment…This is because, culturally, the respect accorded to the elderly is paramount. (Kiata & Kerse, 2004, p. 319)

In contrast, European belief systems are seen as allowing Pākehā elderly a great deal of active agency. Some Pākehā residents may refuse food, care and sometimes medication. This means that health carers have to attempt to reason with the awkward behaviour of these residents (Kiata & Kerse, 2004). In the study, problems that tended to arise were discussed. Pacific Island health carers may have had little or no experience negotiating with unreasonable older people because, in the main, Pacific Island elders are unlikely to refuse care. 'Receiving care remains a major part of a reciprocal relationship between the carer and the cared for in most Pacific [Island] cultures' (Kiata & Kerse, 2004, pp. 320–1).

In contrast to the health carers, residents during the field study explicitly stated that they did not refuse care. Some went on to discuss ethnic differences in caregiving practices. There was talk about the Pacific Island health carers not being as considerate in their care as their Pākehā counterparts. One participant stated that there were differences in care practices between the 'Island and white girls' (Mr C, 80s) but did not expand on this. Another resident said there was not a lot of difference, although some of 'them' (Pacific Islanders) tended to 'be a bit rough' in delivering care (Mrs B, 80s) (Kiata & Kerse, 2004, p. 323).

> How does the cultural and ethnic group you belong to value caring for older people?
> Is there a generation gap between how older people you know expect to be cared for and how you expect to care for them?

A 'generation gap' between the caregivers and residents can occur where views of the world differ substantially between the groups due to age differences. While some elders in residential care have advanced cognitive impairment such

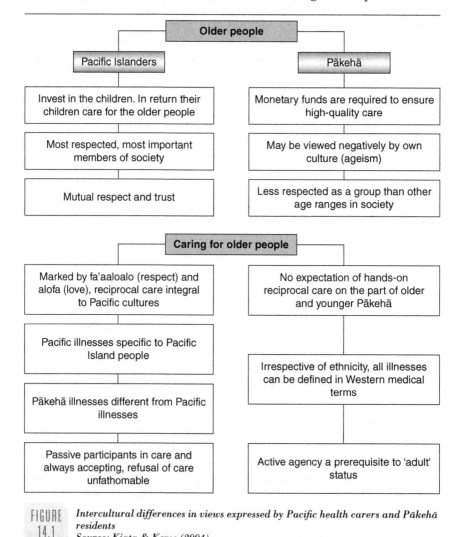

FIGURE 14.1 *Intercultural differences in views expressed by Pacific health carers and Pākehā residents*
Source: Kiata & Kerse (2004)

as dementia, most are aware of the treatment and attitudes they are exposed to during the process of caring. Indeed, one resident expressly negated the idea of old age equating with senility when stating 'because we're old they think we're stupid'. This older woman (Miss E, 90s) suggested that sometimes she gets bored and worries about 'becoming a cabbage'. Another resident scathingly spoke about being patronised by personnel (Kiata & Kerse, 2004, p. 320). Mrs H (90s) had earlier in the day been involved in an interaction with a 'doctor who was talking nonsense this morning, so I talked nonsense back'.

This leads to the lesson that older residents are sensitive to ageist attitudes and are very aware of interactions with and between staff. The views of other ethnic groups about caring for their elders will differ but in general the individualistic active agency of elders in Pākehā culture contrasts with the behaviour of elders from many other ethnic groups, particularly those from New Zealand ethnic minorities (Kiata & Kerse, 2004).

Age-related issues also arise between staff members where age was important to status in some ethnic groups. When a younger caregiver requires help, an older co-worker would not be asked for support because this would be culturally inappropriate. The resident would be left until another person of the same (or similar) generation was available or the resident would be dealt with single-handedly.

> How do you work with your co-workers of different ages and those from different cultural and ethnic groups? What are the issues about what is expected from you in a cultural or ethnic way?

> What are the strategies you use to address imbalances between ethnic groups in care delivery?

FOR REFLECTION

Food as a focus

Food is central to most cultures (Park, 1991) and was one theme that highlighted cultural differences between the Pākehā's and Pacific Islanders' perceptions about taking meals. For example, in Samoan terms, respect for the elderly is epitomised at meal times and becomes evident (to Pākehā) at events such as marriages and funerals (Kiata & Kerse, 2004). 'The elderly are always served first, and the best food is chosen for them. Only when the elders have started to eat can others (even very small children) begin their meals' (Kiata & Kerse, 2004, p. 325). Similarly, the refusal of food when expressly offered is culturally offensive because it illustrates lack of respect and certain foods, particularly delicacies, are perceived in some Pacific Island terms as having certain medicinal properties (Macpherson & Macpherson, 1990).

The right of Pākehā to demand and/or refuse food is in direct contrast to the appropriate behaviour of being a Pacific Island elderly person, who does not expect food at set times. Residents are reported by Pacific health carers to be 'very particular about their food and everything else' and the residents 'usually expect their four-course meals at set times. We have no real control over them' (Carer T, 30s). A health carer bringing in Pacific Island food as a gift for one Pākehā resident's birthday was upset by the negative reaction of the resident, who, it was stated, would not eat the food because it was 'foreign'. Cultural misunderstandings were evident through the very different reactions of the health carer and resident in this situation. The resident did not know and/or did not care that the refusal of this 'gift' was highly offensive and hurtful to the health carer both culturally and personally.

In addition to the health carers views of supplying food as part of practising care, using food as a form of control was also a predominant theme. Certainly, some suggested that food was often used as a bargaining tool to pacify disruptive residents. In one interview, health carers spoke about coping with difficult residents by withholding food. One particularly troublesome resident, who often verbally and physically abused staff, was 'kept in check' by staff withholding food as a punishment. This was achieved by padlocking the refrigerator. In addition, the healthcare assistants dealt with the resident's outbursts by ignoring him for a finite period of time, including meal times. When the resident's behaviour improved, care was resumed and food offered as a reward. These care practices could be loosely interpreted as behavioural techniques in residential care. Application of such techniques should only be used with expert advice from psychologists and dementia behavioural therapists. While these practices may be a common sense solution, withholding of food cannot be condoned as an appropriate practice.

> How is food in the care environment viewed by your cultural and ethnic group?
> How do ethnic and culturally related views of Māori, Asian and North African groups about food differ?
> How do these different views compare to Pākehā norms about food?
> How could these food-related differences impact residents in the care environment?

Caring is physically demanding

There are cultural differences in the way physical care practices are perceived by residents and health carers. A third of health carers in the field study explicitly stated that they were 'more suited to this type of work' than Pākehā and other ethnic groups such as Asians. One spoke in a positive (and Eurocentric) way about the physical prowess of Pacific Island caregivers being suited to this type of work. Some also spoke scornfully about the way that the Pākehā health carers always needed extra assistance when caring for the elderly (Kiata & Kerse, 2004).

These findings can be interpreted in several ways. Because the views of other ethnic groups were not sought, it cannot be said these views are universal; for example, Pākehā health carers may have disagreed with these opinions. It is possible that the health carers contributing to this study were in fact overly confident in not 'ever' requesting assistance with lifting. It is also possible that health carers actively avoided 'demanding' episodes which involved lifting residents.

Figure 14.2 summarises contrasting views of intercultural caring.

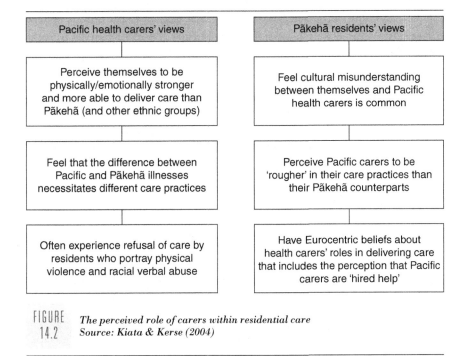

FIGURE 14.2 *The perceived role of carers within residential care*
Source: Kiata & Kerse (2004)

Issues of status

Reciprocal cultural awareness needs to be taken up by both employer and employee in any workplace. As well as issues between health carer and resident, relationships between staff in an ethnically diverse workplace benefit from cultural awareness. For example, among Pacific Island groups, age and societal place are important to status within the community. If a Tongan health carer happened to be employed in a position more 'junior' than another employee who held lower (cultural) status in Tongan society, the ensuing imbalance would sometimes spill over into the work environment. Tension between co-workers resulting from such issues has become apparent to management on more than one occasion.

Racism on the part of residents and staff

In residential care, there is usually a generational difference between health carers and residents. Certainly, residents in New Zealand have often 'lived through the colonial era, when New Zealand was only one of "mother" England's many colonies, and non-Europeans were thought to be inferior to Europeans' (Kiata & Kerse, 2004, p. 322). The term 'being politically correct', that is, not using terms that discriminate and cause offence, such as race-based stereotypes, has little meaning for most residents, as older residents held and expressed racist views during the interviews.

Health carers and nurses are often exposed to verbal racism as well as more covert racist attitudes. Residents may compare cultural difference in terms of 'them and us', with 'us' (those of European (Pākehā) descent) being the 'norm'. For instance, one resident talked about the 'European girls' being all 'very good' as caregivers but the 'darkies' are not so good because they come from different cultures (Mrs H, 90s). In the same vein, another resident suggested that there is not much difference between 'them and us' except in the way physical care was practised (Mrs B, 80s). On the whole, racist comments made by residents were not to be taken seriously by the health carers, or were ignored, thus defusing the situation. What was emphasised most was the need to address the racism as a behavioural problem that 'should not be taken personally'. Whilst exact reasons were not explicitly discussed, the residents may have had a lifetime of experience that may have been devoid of interaction with minority groups. Poor judgement and disinhibition of residents due to illness such as stroke or dementia also may influence this racist behaviour (Kiata & Kerse, 2004).

Views from residents indicated that overall they believed that racist comments were socially acceptable as they had always used stereotypical language. While the residents did not specifically practise racism, Mrs H, who is in her 90s, put this exceedingly well when stating that the Pākehā girls are 'all very good but the darkies are different because they come from different cultures and can be quite bossy; they don't understand us, you see' (Kiata & Kerse, 2004, p. 323). The researchers interpreted this as cultural misunderstanding, rather than misunderstanding due to a language barrier.

> How are issues of racism handled in your current healthcare setting?
> How do the older people you know express views about different cultures and ethnicity that differ from yours?
> Should racist behaviour have to be tolerated because people are old and/or ill?

There was recognition from management that racist behaviour should not be tolerated or condoned, alongside the acknowledgement that this behaviour was often present when the resident had dementia and was not considered 'intentional'. This issue is relevant to all people working in ethnically and culturally diverse settings, and responses to protect workers need to be developed.

Communication

For older people communication through conversing is an important activity and staff members are urged to listen out for the residents' need to talk with other people (Andersson, Pettersson & Sidnevall, 2007; Wadensten, 2005). It has been reported that caregivers need more training in communicating effectively with residents (Carpiac-Claver & Levy-Storms, 2007). Language use effects communication between residents and health carers. While it is important to address residents in a language that they are likely to understand, it was clear that English was the (only) appropriate language to be used at the residence. The reason for implementing this practice came from both residents and employees, who believed that it was rude to speak in languages not understood by all. Further, the English speakers were not sure whether or not they were the topic of conversation or were being ridiculed. This was particularly the case when the Pacific Island health carers punctuated their first-language conversations, such as those in Samoan or Tongan, with peals of laughter.

Sometimes the failure to communicate clearly (in spoken English) led to other methods of communication, for example, body language. One health carer talked about the use of sign language as a way to communicate with residents, some of whom do not speak English well (for example, Asian residents); 'We do a lot of pointing with our fingers and do actions to get our message across to them' (Carer T, 30s). Health carers reported that non-verbal cues were used with success in these situations and that, if you watched and listened, you could generally establish and meet the residents' needs. Misunderstanding and misinterpretation (which are not same) of the English language added to the problem. According to a number of the health carers, misunderstanding sometimes resulted in frustration for the residents and abuse – often based on ethnic lines – followed in a confrontation that resulted in a refusal to accept care (from that caregiver). Misinterpretation had the same outcome but had usually been initiated by a health carer. However, the health carers' language skills were not commented on by the residents.

How can health carers' rights to communicate using their own language be respected without compromising residents' rights to understand what is happening in their 'home'?

Quality of care: significance of cultural differences

Providing a compassionate, caring environment for frail, dependent older people is a challenging task in the complex setting of residential care. The study highlighted a number of elements that may impact on care practices, which could, in turn, affect the quality of care at the residence. There is a need to be more than 'aware' that others come from different ethnic and cultural backgrounds. Cultural safety requires integration of awareness and understanding of others' culturally related needs throughout the delivery of health care. Lack of understanding about the use of particular medicines or ethnocentric cultural views (or both) pertaining to illness (such as speech impediments due to stroke or dementia due to Alzheimer's and Parkinson's disease) will influence the quality of care delivery (Kiata & Kerse, 2004).

Continued learning about how diseases manifest symptoms is a step towards decreasing misinterpretations and misunderstandings. As health carers pointed out, prior to their employment at the residence they had 'no idea about Pākehā sickness' such as Alzheimer's disease and thus had relaxed attitudes towards residents' needs. Their care practices were at that time likely to have reflected this lack of knowledge.

Resistance by residents to health carers' attempts to provide care may also affect outcomes. A number of elderly participants believed that it was detrimental to complain about the ways in which they were cared for. For both health carers and residents, most incidents and accidents occured during the night and morning shifts. Residents were unwilling to bother the staff because the workers were busy. This was further compounded during times of staff shortage by Pacific Island health carers perceiving physical strength as more important than the use of correct lifting techniques, needing two people when moving residents. At other times, dementia-related causes resulted in accidents such as falls and while none of the resident participants had dementia, three did relate experiences of falling because assistance was not called for. Another said that the fall was self-inflicted because it had occurred while attempting to get out of bed unassisted because the call for help remained unanswered. The reasons for residents attempting mobility may have been based on notions of wanting to be self-reliant and maintaining independence.

Residents were, on the other hand, mindful of health carers' needs and all stated the importance of not complaining about their overall treatment 'too much' which could also be related to them feeling vulnerable and dependent upon the health carers (Peri et al., 2008; Ulsperger, 2008). Remaining civil appeared to be an important aspect of the overall relationship the residents had with their health carers. 'One should not complain' said Miss E (90s) 'because the caregivers are always rushing around in order to complete their workload'. This view was echoed by Mrs D, Mrs F and Mrs G (all over 80).

This perception impacts heavily on the social contact the residents have each day. As the majority of residents interviewed had single-bed rooms, being left alone for periods of time, between breakfast and morning tea, for example, will lead to social isolation. Similarly, enforced solitary confinement is compounded by the limited number of visitors that residents receive. For, as one of the women mentioned above succinctly stated, 'everyone is so busy you know'. The term 'everyone' includes the health carers. Two residents in single-bed rooms spoke about the impact of conditions that were not medically treatable, such as the loss of adequate sight or gnarled fingers due to arthritis. These conditions led to a reduction in activities such as reading and knitting.

Conclusion

This field study highlights the need to better understand the care environment from the perspective of both health carers and the residents to whom they provide care. Values and views of ageing can influence the way care is delivered. Understanding the expectations of older residents can make it easier for health carers to meet those expectations. The reality of knowing the subtleties of 'your own' and/or 'other' cultural protocols is often overlooked. What may seem to be the norm to Pākehā may be totally inappropriate for some people from the

Pacific Islands and other cultures, and vice versa. For example, asking for help from an elder is socially acceptable, indeed, often expected, in Pākehā culture. However, in some Pacific cultures, asking for an older health carer's help to lift a resident is culturally unacceptable due to the concept of 'respecting one's elders'.

While learning about culture can help understanding factors such as time, or staff issues, cultural constraints can interfere with how caring is delivered and received. The autonomy of the resident has to be balanced against the resident's level of ability and safety issues are considered at all times. This balance between the practical tasks involved in completing caregiving effectively in culturally safe ways deserves consideration in the workplace by all involved in residential care.

Another factor that could affect care is that the caregiving role is under-valued and underpaid in our society. Our study agrees with findings of other research that caregiving often involves limited on-the-job training and low pay. These factors do not match with the importance of the work that health carers are expected to carry out (Burns et al., 1999).

This chapter points out that there needs to be cultural awareness when car-ing for people living and working in residential care. Working towards positive outcomes of good care practices, for both residents and health carers, means developing respect for and awareness of the needs of minority residents, resi-dents' families, health carers and management within the context of their cul-ture. Yet, both internationally and in New Zealand, there remains a gap in the research about intercultural care practices – both in general terms, and specifi-cally in terms of how care practices work effectively, or not, across cultural and ethnic boundaries. In the following practice exercises you can discuss some of these intercultural issues.

FOR REFLECTION

The exercises below may be useful when reflecting on the material in this chapter.

Age

How do you think ageism might affect the practical delivery of care? Examples:

> Views on age-related tasks within and between culturally and ethnically diverse groups may affect cooperation and 'helping out' among health carers.

> Older health carers may resent the easy time that they perceive younger workers to be having.

> If the older person has an ageist view, this can affect the way they portray themselves to their health carers and other health professionals.

Behaviour

Consider active agency and its affect on the reciprocal relationship needed for successful caregiving. What do you consider to be appropriate behaviour for people working and living in residential care?

Examples:

> How could particular cultural patterns of Pacific Islanders' behaviour, for example, singing, clapping and laughing loudly, be considered inappropriate by management?

> How do cultural variations on what is considered appropriate behaviour in residential care impact on the way residents are cared for?

> How are care practices impacted on by culturally related misunderstandings between health carers and those they care for?

Racism

How do culturally and ethnically diverse health carers deal with racism from older, usually Pākehā, residents?

Examples:

> How is racist behaviour displayed by older people ignored or accepted in a care setting? Is this behaviour seen as acceptable because people are old and/or ill?

> How do racist remarks affect the way in which health carers interact with, and care for, residents?

> Does management tolerate racist behaviour too much at times?

Communication

When communicating, how does the use of different languages in a residential care context work? Comment on whether language is a barrier to, or a promoter of, communication.

Examples:

> Could the use of 'foreign' languages by health carers make residents feel uncomfortable and that they are being 'talked about'?

> How do policies such as spoken English only policies produce resentment on the part of non-English first language speakers?

> Can limited spoken English be a way for health carers to avoid doing extra work or result in extra work?

References

Andersson, I., Pettersson, E. & Sidnevall, B. (2007). Daily life after moving into a care home – experiences from older people, relatives and contact persons. *Journal of Clinical Nursing*, 16(9), 1712–18.

Boyd, M., Connolly, M., Kerse, N., Foster, S., von Randow, M., Lay-Yee, R.… Walters-Puttick, S. (2009). *Changes in aged care residents' characteristics and dependency in Auckland 1988 to 2008*. Auckland: Freemasons' Department of Geriatric Medicine, University of Auckland.

Burns, J., Dwyer, M., Lambie, H. & Lynch, J. (1999). *Homecare workers: A case study of a female occupation*. Wellington: Ministry of Women's Affairs.

Carpiac-Claver, M. L. & Levy-Storms, L. (2007). In a manner of speaking: Communication between nurse aides and older adults in long-term care settings. *Health Communication*, 22(1), 59–67.

Denzin, N. (ed.). (1994). *The art and politics of interpretation: Handbook of qualitative research*. London: Sage.

Department of Health. (1988). *The care, mis-care and abuse of the elderly*. Wellington: Department of Health.

Diamond, T. (1992). *Making gray gold: Narratives of nursing home care*. Chicago: University of Chicago Press.

Foner, N. (1995). *The caregiving dilemma: Work in an American Nursing Home*. Berkeley: University of California Press.

Fry, C. (2000). Culture, age, and subjective well-being: Health, functionality, and the infrastructure of eldercare in comparative perspective. *Journal of Family Issues*, *21*(6), 751–76.

Gallant, M. P., Sptize, G. & Grove, J. G. (2010). Chronic illness self-care and the family lives of older adults: A synthetic review across four ethnic groups. *Journal of Cross-Cultural Gerontology*, *25*(1), 21–42.

Kiata, L. & Kerse, N. (2004). Intercultural residential care in New Zealand. *Journal of Qualitative Health Research*, *14*(3), 313–27 (March).

Macpherson, C. & Macpherson, L. (1990). *Samoan medical belief and practice*. Auckland: Auckland University Press.

Ministry of Health. (2013). *Showcasing aged-care nursing*. Wellington: Ministry of Health. Retrieved 21 November 2014 from http://www.health.govt.nz

North Shore Old People's Welfare Council. (1969). Seminar on the problems of the elderly. North Shore Old People's Welfare Council, Auckland.

Organisation for Economic Cooperation and Development. (1996). *Ageing in OECD Countries: A critical policy challenge*. Paris: Organisation for Economic Cooperation and Development.

Park, J. (ed.). (1991). *Ladies a plate: Change and continuity in the lives of New Zealand women*. Auckland: Auckland University Press.

Peri, K., Fanslow, J., Hand, J. & Parsons, J. (2008). *Elder abuse and neglect: Exploration of risk and protective factors*. Wellington: Families Commission.

Peri, K., Kerse, N., Robinson, E., Parson, M., Parsons, J. & Latham, N. (2008). Does functionally based activity make a difference to health status and mobility? A randomised controlled trial in residential care facilities (The Promoting Independent Living Study; PILS). *Age and Ageing, 37*, 57–63. doi:10.1093/ageing/afm135

Sevenhuijsen, S. R. L. (1998). *Citizenship and the ethics of care: Feminist considerations on justice, morality and politics*. London: Routledge.

Tarlow, B. (1996). Caring: A negotiated process that varies. In S. Gordon, P. Benner & N. Noddings (eds) *Caregiving, readings in knowledge, practice, ethics and politics* (pp. 76–92). Philadelphia: University of Pennsylvania Press.

Ulsperger, J. S. (2008). The social dynamics of elder care: Rituals of bureaucracy and physical neglect in nursing homes. *Sociological Spectrum, 28*, 357–88.

Wadensten, B. (2005). The content of morning time conversations between nursing home staff and residents. *Journal of Clinical Nursing, 14*(2), 84–9.

Wilkinson, T., Kiata, L., Peri, K., Robinson, E. & Kerse, N. (2012). Quality of life for older people in residential care is related to connectedness, willingness to enter care, and co-residents. *Australasian Journal on Ageing, 31*(1), 52–5. doi:10.1111/j.1741-6612.2010.00503.x

Wilson, G. (2000). *Understanding old age: Critical and global perspectives*. London: Sage.

Acknowledgements

The authors would like to thank the Health Research Council of New Zealand who provided financial support for this study to be undertaken. We would also like to thank the health care and residents of the residential setting chosen for this study for sharing their time and narratives. This study would not have been possible if the participants had not been willing to share their perceptions. Thanks are extended to the management for allowing ready access and for clarifying background information on the residence setting. We would also like to thank Professor Julie Park, Dr Sally Abel, Associate Professor Stephen Buetow, Dr Vivienne Adair, Junior Tutagalevao and Dr Tamasailau Suaalii-Sauni for their contributions, which led to this chapter being written. Material presented in this chapter is also published in an article in the *Journal of Qualitative Health Research* (Kiata & Kerse, 2004). Text and artwork are reprinted by permission of SAGE Publications.

15 Sex, gender and sexual orientation

Sallie Greenwood

Learning objectives

Having studied this chapter, you will be able to:

- become familiar with the distinction between the concepts of 'sex' and 'gender';

- explore the dualism of male and female, its presumed 'naturalness' and its relationship to sexual expression;

- reflect on the discrimination that can occur when stereotypical ideas of sex, gender and sexual orientation are applied within health and social care.

Key terms and concepts

- androgynous

- biphobia

- heterosexism

- homophobia

- intersex

- sexual orientation

Introduction

This chapter is concerned with sex and gender, the distinctions between them, and what is assumed about how a person expresses their sexuality. The intention of this chapter is to bring some of the unconscious assumptions about sex, gender and sexual orientation into focus, and to challenge some of the ideological beliefs that underpin them. Why these terms are important and what they have to do with cultural safety is explored.

What do people see when they look in the mirror or when they look at other people? Perhaps age and ethnicity, perhaps also gender. They may or may not see aspects of the sexed body. Inevitably assumptions are made – it is the way minds work in order to manage the volume of information that confronts people in everyday life and work. When meeting new people, aspects of their identity that are immediately visible are registered. It's done unconsciously. It's noticed if they are big or small, thin or fat, light or dark, male or female, old or young, and so on. Language situates these aspects as dualisms – they are this or that – which enables people to categorise things in a simple fashion. Yet, there is much more diversity in the world.

It seems that, in order to feel comfortable communicating with others, people need to 'know' some of their attributes because these determine the cultural rules of right behaviour. Interactions with people change according to relative ages, genders and ethnicities. Each of these attributes also intersects with the others so that, for example, an older person who is male is interacted with differently to an older person who is female. Further differences complicate this when we include ethnicity. Sometimes people can get it wrong and then attempt to remedy their mistakes.

In the unconscious checklist of attributes, gender is often synonymous with the sexed body, such that female is synonymous with feminine and male with masculine. If the person's sex is indeterminate or androgynous, people are unsure how to proceed in case conventions are breached; they feel uncomfortable.

A word about language

This chapter uses the shorthand term 'LBGT' for gay, lesbian, bisexual and transgender people and some writers cited in this chapter use the political term 'queer' to include LBGT people. Māori and Pacific peoples have their own languages to describe transgender, gay and lesbian people; terms which carry different cultural meanings. Some of the terms used are Fa'faffine, Whakawahine, and Tangata ira Tane for transgender people (Clark et al., 2014) or Takatāpui (Te Awekotuku, 1991) for gay and lesbian people.

> ❯ Can you recall a time when you saw a person whose sex/gender was unclear to you?
> ❯ If so, reflect on the feelings you experienced and how you responded (internally) to them.

FOR
REFLECTION

A history of sex and gender

The terms 'sex' and 'gender' are often used interchangeably, yet many writers distinguish them in terms of sex being associated with the biological body and gender the more socially constructed aspects of identity. If gender is socially constructed, it must be dependent on cultural understandings such that what is deemed appropriate behaviour for males and females is determined by the culture one grows up in. Sex on the other hand is sometimes understood to be immutable and outside of culture because it is biologically determined. However, this is an oversimplification of the natural diversity and changeability of human bodies.

Until the late 1950s the term 'sex' was used almost exclusively to talk about men and women. This was as true in the academic literature as in the general public. Muehlenhard and Peterson (2011) conducted a search of the psychological literature and found 6756 results during or before 1960 that used the term sex to talk about males and females and only 32 that talked about gender. This reflects the prevailing assumption of the time regarding the naturalness of sexed behaviour. The earliest mention of gender was by John Money and colleagues in 1955 (Money, 1994) who researched people they referred to as hermaphrodites and who we would now refer to as intersex – people born with the sexual characteristics of both males and females. Money was interested in their anatomical and physiological make up, as well as their childhood socialisation and psychological aspects of gender. In particular, he was interested in how gendered identity had been socialised and later expressed. Although Money's work heralded new understandings about sex and gender, it was still very much grounded in the cultural expressions of gender of the time.

Since Money's early work, the sex/gender distinction has become increasingly important for researchers and social movements. For the feminist movement it prefigured the phrase 'biology is not destiny' – an idea that was written into a popular play by Renée performed in New Zealand called *Born to Clean* – a parody on the cultural assumptions about women's work. Distinguishing between sex and gender provided opportunities for feminists to argue that the division of labour, where men worked outside the home in paid employment and women worked inside the home and undertook all the child care, was artificial. Anthropologist Gail Rubin (1975) argued that gender was more about the suppression of the similarities between men and women than about natural hardwired differences between them and further, that such suppression served the divisions of labour seen in societies.

In 1990 Judith Butler wrote her book entitled *Gender Trouble* in which she argues that gender was a performance; something that is done, not something that is. In using the term 'performance' Butler did not mean that the way people express themselves in a gendered way is trivial or unreal only that it is a socially constructed way of being. If gender is a performance – the way that people 'do' gender reflects the culture in which they have come to know themselves as gendered subjects. Some cultures construct a greater diversity of gendered expressions than others but their expressions are still recognisable within their own culture. Only when the gendered performance does not seem to fit does it cause discomfort in those observing it. People may have moved somewhat from the imperative that boys mustn't cry, yet seeing a man crying still evokes different thoughts and feelings than when a woman cries.

Consider how you 'do' gender and what kinds of behaviours define you in terms of being masculine, feminine or indeterminate.

Some people may feel resistance to Butler's ideas about performance and believe that the way gender is expressed is informed largely by the physical sex, genetic make up and hormonal activity. This leaves at least two views about sex/gender: the *realist* view that sees biology as playing the major part in and the *constructionist* view that people are largely culturally determined. Most people would agree that there are some biological differences between male and female bodies. There are the obvious ones associated with women's capacity to carry and give birth to children but is this a defining difference? How sex/ gender is understood is important for health because there do appear to be some epidemiological differences (Doull et al., 2010). There is, for example, evidence (see Parker, Kalasky & Proctor, 2010) that there are important differences in cardiovascular disease processes and prognosis.

However, whilst Hammarstrom and Annandale (2012) agree that sociocultural and biological factors are important, they argue that the differences have been exaggerated and cite Patsopoulos and Ioannidis (2007) who suggest that most of the claims made about genetic sex differences cannot be verified. Even if there is assent to the view that sex/gender has some genetic components, knowledge of epigenetics shows that genes can be turned on and off depending on the environment and experiences of the person. So how influential genes are in producing sex/gender is unclear.

In addition to the apparent differences between males and females, there are also a vast range of differences within bodies labelled 'male' and bodies labelled 'female' as well as between them. Additionally, there are many bodies that do not fit neatly into either view – people who are intersex, transgender or transsexual.

Discrimination

When talking about cultural safety, discrimination matters very much because people are often discriminated against when they don't fit preconceived ideas about what is 'normal' sex, gender and sexual orientation. Discrimination can be in the form of bullying (Collier, Bos & Sandford, 2013) and other forms of violence, exclusion from social activities, or in the limitations imposed on health care. In New Zealand young people who identify as transgender or are unsure of their gender are significantly more at risk of violence, bullying and mental health issues as a result of their isolation (Clark et al., 2014). Pitts et al. (2009) find that transgender people in Australia and New Zealand who had experienced discrimination were, not surprisingly, more likely to suffer from depression. Yet, they are less likely to be treated in general medical or community-based settings for mental health or other medical conditions because health professionals believe that they require specialist psychiatric care (Drescher, Cohen-Kettenis & Winter, 2012). This is so even when their conditions are not related to being transgender.

Research has shown that LGBT people are less likely to receive appropriate health care (Irwin, 2007), in part because they are assumed to be heterosexual by health professionals, and also because a third do not disclose their sexual orientation to these professionals for fear of discrimination (Chapman, Zappia & Shields, 2012; Neville & Henrickson, 2006).

Sexed bodies

It is clear that culture and ethnicity produce different kinds of bodies. When comparing the muscle development of sportspeople in New Zealand 50 years ago with the sportspeople of today, it is easy to see that bodies are influenced by their social context. Additionally, '[e]thnicity is well-recognized to incorporate a variety of different components of phenotype, including variation in DNA sequence or expression, physiology, behaviour, lifestyle and values/perceptions' (Wells, 2012, p. 15).

International sporting bodies appear to have taken a rather narrow view of what constitutes a normal body for the purposes of sport. In the 1960s women competing in the Olympics, who were considered too masculine, were subjected to the humiliation of having to walk naked in front of physicians to prove that they were female (Cooky & Dworkin, 2013; Park, 2012). From 1968 to

1998, adopting advances in scientific testing, the International Olympic Committee (IOC) instituted mandatory sex testing in women's sport (Elias et al., 2000) using chromosome tests. These tests proved to be problematic because, as chromosomes vary, biological sex is a very complex thing to determine. Despite the difficulties, the IOC still reserves the right to test competitors whose sex/gender is 'suspicious' (Cooky & Dworkin, 2013).

Muehlenhard and Peterson (2011), in their paper looking at the history and current implication of the sex/gender distinction, advise not to confuse social construction with the concept of socialisation. They argue that it is 'societies [that] create categories of sex – such as male and female – and assign individuals to each (p. 801).' When people do not appear to fit easily into the predetermined categories, ways are found to change them so that they do fit. This can be chemically or surgically. Alternatively people 'can be encouraged to keep their differences hidden; or... treated as aberrant, unfortunate individuals who were born with a defect; that is, the problem can be attributed to individuals rather than to society's narrow categories'. Society can then continue to believe that the categories created are natural and that people fit into them with no trouble.

Gender

Though many people take gender for granted, there are also a number of people who experience the dualism of male or female as limited in describing their experience of themselves. There are people in many countries, including Australia and New Zealand, who 'substantially challenge gender expectations' (Pyne, 2014, p. 1). 'Gender non-conforming' or 'gender variance' are terms that encompass a range of experience. For example, there are people who are comfortable with their biological sex but who express themselves in non-conforming gendered behaviours. Others may completely reject the terms boy and girl and see no reason to choose; some may identify with a different gender to their sex and may later go on to become transsexual (Pyne, 2014).

In the past these young people would have been treated as pathological and subjected to various attempts at a 'cure'. The DSM-5, the latest version of the *Diagnostic and Statistical Manual of Mental Disorders* (DSM) (American Psychiatric Association, 2013a) used to diagnose mental illness, has a classification of 'gender dysphoria' which replaces the previous classification of 'gender identity disorder'. It is said 'to better characterize the experiences of affected children, adolescents, and adults' (American Psychiatric Association, 2013b).

Conversely, critics have said this is a matter of semantics that continues to pathologise the diversity of gendered experience.

Despite the pathologisation and stigmatisation experienced by transgender people, Pyne (2014) submits that there has been a paradigm shift, marked by terms such as 'gender independent', in the way that we understand gender now compared to 30 or 40 years ago. She cites the work of various social movements such as feminism, queer liberation and transgender rights, along with compelling evidence from animal biologists that there are more than two sexes in the biological world, as being responsible for this shift.

Therefore, it would seem that there are areas of enlightenment while at the same time an adherence to traditional ideas about gender. For example, it is still difficult to buy a gender neutral birthday card for anyone, and particularly for a child, where the norm continues to be highly stereotypically gendered with graphics such as puppies and pink dresses for girls and footballs and cars for boys.

In terms of professional engagement with young people who are gender independent, transgender, transsexual, lesbian and gay, young and old may still struggle to be respected and included in all of life's opportunities. As long as narrow and limiting categories continue to inform our reality, we will not see the diversity of experience of the people we come into contact with.

Anne

Practice example 1

Anne is a 54-year-old woman. She has short, grey hair and a rounded body shape. She wears trousers, shirts and flat serviceable shoes. Sometimes in shops she is addressed as 'Sir' before the sales assistant notices that she may have breasts and doesn't have signs of facial hair. Outwardly this does not appear to concern Anne but in fact it does upset her. She positively identifies as female and has no wish to be seen as a man. Being a woman is important to Anne although she does not represent herself stereotypically. When Anne attends her local general practice for her regular smear, Carol, the new practice nurse who is going to undertake the procedure, is unsure about how she should approach health promotion with Anne around sexual health. She wonders if Anne is still sexually active and if Anne identifies as lesbian or heterosexual. Carol is also concerned that she might offend Anne by enquiring about her sexuality.

FOR REFLECTION

> If you were Carol how would you engage with Anne in a health-promoting relationship?

> What are the social and professional influences that inform your thinking?

> How would you feel if you were asked to prove your biological sex because your physical and/or gendered expression did not conform to the views commonly held by those who had the power to limit your behaviour?

Sexual orientation

The term 'sex' being associated with biology is also a term used to infer sexual behaviour or 'having sex'. Despite changing attitudes and more openness in many Western countries around expressions of sexuality, the dominant assumption of heterosexuality is still prevalent. In this frame, males are masculine, females are feminine and they 'have sex' with each other. Thus sex, gender and sexuality are assumed to be in 'normal' biological alignment. There is a much greater acceptance of homosexuality but this tends to be accompanied by assumptions that reproduce heterosexual difference (Drescher, 2010). Gay men are assumed to be 'feminine' and lesbian women more 'masculine'. Paradoxically it is again assumed that they will partner with someone whose gender reflects their sex in normative ways. Thus gay and lesbian couples are sometimes viewed as mimicking heterosexuality. However, what persists in the imagination is that someone who looks like a woman and acts stereotypically like a woman will be heterosexual. This assumption is made by health and social practice professionals as well as the general public. When these assumptions are made, the gay or lesbian person has to make a choice whether to go along with the assumption and hide their reality or to correct the assumption and risk prejudice.

Until 1973 homosexuality was considered a psychiatric disorder in need of treatment. It was then changed in the DSM II to 'sexual orientation disturbance' with the implication that someone who identified as homosexual, but was 'disturbed' by it, could be diagnosed. The stigmatisation remained and in the DSM III the term was changed to 'ego dystonic homosexuality' and eventually dropped altogether during a later change. Nevertheless the stigma of mental illness is still associated by some with homosexuality because of its long historical connection with the DSM, despite it no longer being classified as such.

How sex, gender and sexual orientation is viewed intersects with ethnicity in the same way as it intersects with age, religion or spirituality. Whilst there may be an increasing acceptance of homosexuality in the young, older people are more likely to be assumed to be heterosexual due to ageist assumptions. As the population increasingly ages and more elderly people are cared for in nursing homes, this will become more of an issue (Kimmel, 2014). Currently it is difficult for some care staff to accept that older people are sexual beings let alone that they are sexual with people of the same sex. The stigma of being considered 'sick' remains for many older gay and lesbian people, and also makes it difficult for them to be open about their relationships.

Kevin

Kevin is an 89-year-old gay man who has lived with his partner for over 40 years. He was a high court judge for a number of years and is very conservative. He and his partner have not been publically open about their sexuality because, when they met, their sexuality was illegal. Kevin's partner, James, was hospitalised in a psychiatric ward when he was in his early 20s because of his homosexuality and subjected to electroconvulsive treatment. Kevin has been admitted to the rehabilitation ward of a private hospital following a cerebrovascular accident and you are the registered nurse responsible for his care.

Kevin's rehabilitation is going to take a long time and the couple have decided that they should relocate to a retirement village so that they can receive support with Kevin's care when he is well enough.

FOR REFLECTION

> As you engage in a relationship with Kevin and James, what are the things you need to consider about their experiences, and your own attitudes and preconceptions?

> What are your thoughts and feelings about older people's sexual expression?

LBGT refugees from countries where homosexuality is forbidden often experience added difficulties in the country that they flee to. 'Five [countries] maintain the death penalty for male homosexual acts and four for sexual acts between women' (Jordon, 2009, p. 166). When LBGT refugees seek asylum in other countries they have to navigate a refugee system that was not designed for their experiences. As Jordon argues: 'The refugee system, implicitly and explicitly, evaluates applicants against expected trajectories of *refugee flight* and against Western narratives of LGBT identities, *coming out, or gender identity dysphoria*' (p.166, emphasis in the original). The journeys for LBGT refugees can often be very different, as they try to hide their identity in their country of origin, and then as they make their way out under difficult circumstances

In this instance Jordon is discussing the Canadian system but there is no reason to suppose that it is different in New Zealand. Queer migrants are negotiating sexual difference, ethnic difference and migratory experience within a complex political climate with regard to the movement of people between countries.

Conclusion

The stigma associated with transgender identity can make adjustment difficult, especially for teenagers, which may sometimes result in young people being referred to psychiatric or psychological services. The traditional psychiatric method of working with children and adults whose gender does not conform to societal expectations, such as using cognitive behavioural therapy and psychodynamic approaches has, according to Malpas (2011), been largely unsuccessful in supporting them. In contrast Malpas discusses an affirmative approach which sees gender as existing on a fluid spectrum and has the aim of de-stigmatising and normalising people's experiences. It requires a *both/and* stance rather than an *either/or* stance, recognising and affirming the person whilst understanding the limits of the gender binary in contemporary society. Working with the family/whānau involves 'protection and acceptance, adaptation, and nurturing' (Malpas, p. 457). This approach requires flexibility on the part of the professional working with the family/whānau, as each member comes to terms with what it means for themselves, their child, sibling or parent to identify their gender differently to social conventions.

Health and social practice professionals are in key positions to advocate for greater awareness and openness to the diversity of human life. We might say that it is an ethical imperative and as nurse Tina Donnelly (2011, p. 13) argues, 'we have to challenge homophobia, biphobia and heterosexism in the workplace whenever we encounter it'.

Psychologist Laurence Kirmayer (2013, p. 370) reminds us that cultural safety includes a number of strategies:

> recognizing the histories and current contexts that structure inequality; embodying and enacting difference, mutual respect, and serious but playful engagement; and especially, an explicit emphasis on tolerance of not-knowing as a bracketing of professional expertise, a realistic appraisal of limitations, and an ethical stance before the face of the other.

Kirmayer goes on to argue that neutrality or ignoring difference can be 'the most biased and provocative stance imaginable'. Here I am reminded of Irihapeti Ramsden's (1992) imperative that to be culturally safe we must treat all people *regardful* of their differences to us. That has to include the differences we do not know about because people do not feel safe to disclose them (Chapman, Zappia & Shields, 2012). Therefore, our 'tolerance of not-knowing' and 'bracketing of professional expertise' or letting go of reliance on professional knowledge, become our greatest strengths as culturally safe practitioners.

FOR REFLECTION

> Look at popular magazine advertisements. How are sex and gender used to sell products? Which products use stereotypical images of gender and which use models whose sex/gender is ambiguous? Who is the intended audience?

> What is the importance of distinguishing between sex and gender?

> Thinking about your responses to people that you see in the community, what do you assume about their sex/gender/sexual orientation? What are the aspects you consider as you make the assessment? Are you assuming that their gender is reflective of their sexed body, for example?

> How might heterosexist attitudes of health and social practice professionals impact on LGBT people's health-seeking behaviours?

> How do you think you might work affirmatively with a young person and their family/whānau in relation to the young person's gender-independent position?

> How do you think you might work affirmatively with parents whose baby is intersex?

> How would you work with a refugee who has come from a culture where their sex/gender/sexual orientation transgressed their country's laws?

References

American Psychiatric Association. (2013a). *Diagnostic and statistical manual of mental disorders* (5th edn.). Washington: American Psychiatric Association.

American Psychiatric Association. (2013b). *Gender dysphoria.* Washington: American Psychiatric Publishing. Retrieved 21 November 2014 from http://www.dsm5.org/documents/gender%20dysphoria%20fact%20sheet.pdf

Butler, J. (1990). *Gender trouble: Feminism and the subversion of identity.* New York: Routledge.

Chapman, R., Zappia, T. & Shields, L. (2012). An essay about health professionals' attitudes to lesbian, gay, bisexual and transgender parents seeking healthcare for their children. *Scandinavian Journal of Caring Sciences, 26,* 333–9. doi: 10.1111/j.1471–6712.2011.00938.x

Clark, T. C., Lucassen, M. F. G., Bullen, P., Denny, S. J., Fleming, T. M., Robinson, E. M. & Rossen, F. V. (2014). The health and well-being of transgender high school students: Results from the New Zealand adolescent health survey (Youth'12). *Journal of Adolescent Health 55,* 93–9. Retrieved 11 July 2014 from http://www.jahonline.org

Collier, K. L., Bos, H. M. W. & Sandford, T. G. M. (2013). Homophobic name-calling among secondary school students and its implications for mental health. *Journal of Youth Adolescence, 42,* 363–75.

Cooky, C. & Dworkin, S. L. (2013). Policing the boundaries of sex: A critical examination of gender verification and the Caster Semenya controversy. *Journal of Sex Research, 50*(2), 103–11. doi: 10.1080/00224499.2012.725488

Donnelly, T. (2011). Embracing diversity is a source of strength to our profession. *Nursing Standard, 25*(22), 12–13.

Doull, M., Runnels, V. E., Tudiver, S. & Boscoe, M. (2010). Appraising the evidence: Applying sex- and gender-based analysis (SGBA) to Cochrane systematic reviews on cardiovascular disease. *Journal of Women's Health, 19*(5), 997–1003. doi: 10.1089=jwh.2009.1626

Drescher, J. (2010). Queer diagnoses: Parallels and contrasts in the history of homosexuality, gender variance, and the Diagnostic and Statistical Manual (DSM). *Archives of Sexual Behavior, 39,* 427–60. doi: 10.1007/s10508-009-9531-5

Drescher, J., Cohen-Kettenis, P. & Winter, S. (2012). Minding the body: Situating gender identity diagnosis in the ICD-11. *International Review of Psychiatry, 24*(6), 568–77. doi: 10.3109/09540261.2012.741575

Elias, L. J., Ljungqvist, A., Ferguson-Smith, M., Simpson, J. L., Genel, M. & Carlson, A. S. (2000). Gender verification of female athletes. *Genetics in Medicine, 2,* 249–54.

Hammarstrom, A. & Annandale, E. (2012). A conceptual muddle: An empirical analysis of the use of 'sex' and 'gender' in 'gender-specific medicine' journals. *PLoS ONE, 7*(4), 1–8. Retrieved 10 July 2014 from http://www.plosone.org

Irwin, L. (2007). Homophobia and heterosexism: Implications for nursing and nursing practice. *Australian Journal of Advanced Nursing, 25,* 70–6.

Jordon, S. H. (2009). Un/Convention(al) refugees: Contextualizing the accounts of refugees facing homophobic or transphobic persecution. *Refuge, 26*(2), 165–82. Retrieved 11 July 2014 from http://pi.library.yorku.ca/ojs/index.php/refuge/article/viewPDFInterstitial/32086/29332

Kimmel, D. (2014). Lesbian, gay, bisexual, and transgender aging concerns. *Clinical Gerontologist, 37*(1), 49–63. doi:10.1080/07317115.2014.847310

Kirmayer, L. J. (2013). Embracing uncertainty as a path to competence: Cultural safety, empathy, and alterity in clinical training. *Culture, Medicine and Psychiatry, 37,* 365–72. doi 10.1007/s11013-013-9314-2

Malpas, J. (2011). Between pink and blue: A multi-dimensional family approach to gender nonconforming children and their families. *Family Process, 50*(4), 453–70. Retrieved 11 July 2014 from http://www.onlinelibrary.wiley.com/journal/famp

Money, J. (1994). The concept of gender identity disorder in childhood and adolescence after 39 years. *Journal of Sex & Marital Therapy, 20*(3), 163–77.

Muehlenhard, C. L. & Peterson, Z. D. (2011). Distinguishing between sex and gender: History, current conceptualisation, and implications. *Sex Roles, 64,* 791–803. doi 10.1007/s11199-011-9932-5

Neville, S. & Henrickson, M. (2006). Perceptions of lesbian, gay and bisexual people of primary healthcare services. *Journal of Advanced Nursing, 55,* 407–15.

Park, A. (2012). Woman enough? Inside the controversial world of Olympic gender testing. *Time, 180*(1), 19. Retrieved 11 July 2014 from http://www.time.com/time/

Parker, B. A., Kalasky, M. J. & Proctor, D. N. (2010). Evidence for sex differences in cardiovascular aging and adaptive responses to physical activity. *European Journal of Applied Physiology, 110*, 235–46. doi 10.1007/s00421–010–1506–7

Pitts, M. K., Couch, M., Mulcare, H., Croy, S. & Mitchell, A. (2009). Transgender people in Australia and New Zealand: Health, well-being and access to health services. *Feminism & Psychology, 19*(4), 475–95. doi: 10.1177/0959353509342771

Pyne, J. (2014). Gender independent kids: A paradigm shift in approaches to gender non-conforming children. *Canadian Journal of Human Sexuality, 23*(1), 1–8. doi:10.3138/cjhs.23.1.CO1

Ramsden, I. (1992) *Kawa Whakaruruhau: Guidelines for nursing and midwifery education.* Wellington: Nursing Council of New Zealand.

Rubin, G. & Reiter, R. R. (1975). *The traffick in women: Notes on the "political economy" of sex.* New York: Monthly Review Press.

Te Awekotuku, N. (1991). *Mana wahine Māori. Selected writings on Māori women's art, culture, and politics.* Auckland: New Women's Press.

Wells, J. C. K. (2012). Ethnic variability in adiposity, thrifty phenotypes and cardiometabolic risk: Addressing the full range of ethnicity, including those of mixed ethnicity. *Obesity Reviews, 13*(Supplement 2), 14–29. doi: 10.1111/j.1467–789X.2012.01034.x

16 Māori health
MĀORI- AND WHĀNAU-CENTRED PRACTICE

Denise Wilson and Huhana Hickey

Learning obectives

Having studied this chapter, you will be able to:

- critically discuss the need for Māori- and whānau-centred services;

- describe the importance of whānau ora for improving access and use of health services by Māori and whānau;

- apply the principles of culturally responsive and whānau-centred practice to working with Māori and their whānau;

- develop strategies for working with Māori, whānau and communities for optimal health service experiences, and to improve their health outcomes.

Key terms and concepts

- equity

- hauora

- inequities

- rights

- tino rangatiratanga

- whānau ora

Introduction

The right to experience health and well-being by accessing necessary determinants of health, and encounter quality health services is embedded in the principles of social justice, equity and rights. For Māori, their rights extend beyond the human rights afforded to everyone living in Aotearoa, to include Te Tiriti o Waitangi/ Treaty of Waitangi ('the Treaty') and, more recently, the

United Nation's *Declaration on the Rights of Indigenous Peoples* (signed by New Zealand in 2010). Article 24.2 states that: 'Indigenous individuals have an equal right to the enjoyment of the highest attainable standard of physical and mental health' (United Nations , 2008, p. 9). Article 3 of the Treaty affirms Māori, as tangata whenua, the same (equal) rights as others living in Aotearoa, which includes health (Durie, 1998). Moreover, the Treaty guarantees tino rangatiratanga – the right to control their life.

Māori and their whānau live with significant disparities and inequities in their health status and health outcomes compared to other groups living in Aotearoa, despite their rights to equality in health and self-determination. They are subjected to a 'one size fits all' style of health services that invariably does not accommodate their health or cultural needs (Wilson & Barton, 2012). Māori are most likely to:

- have poor access to necessary determinants of health (such as having socio-economic resources);
- experience chronic health conditions (Robson, Cormack & Cram, 2007);
- not have their health needs met (Ministry of Health, 2012);
- face discrimination (Harris et al., 2012);
- die before 'old age' (Ministry of Health, 2010a).

Yet, despite their right to determine and control decisions about their life, health and well-being, these are generally made for them by health service policy makers, planners and health professionals.

Optimal health outcomes means that health services and healthcare professionals need to deliver culturally safe and appropriate services to Māori and their whānau. Accurate and adequate information, along with access to quality services, are crucial so they can benefit from what health services offer. Māori and their whānau require healthcare professionals to give sufficient and accurate information about their health and any conditions they may have. Interventions and services should also be appropriate for their life circumstances and delivered so that they understand information provided to make informed decisions. This also includes information about additional health and/or social services needed, particularly Māori- or whānau-centred services within their community. In this chapter we provide an overview of Māori world views and the importance of whānau, followed by the development of whānau ora. We then explore whānau-centred practice, and strategies for working with Māori, their whānau and their communities.

Māori world views and whānau

Health is a sociocultural construction, informed by the particular world views that people have, and influenced by their life experiences. The Māori concept of health – hauora – is wellness focused and grounded within a Māori world view. This view of health contrasts with the ill-health rhetoric that is often synonymous with being Māori. Māori world views, similar to other indigenous people's world views, are holistic, grounded in whakapapa (genealogy), wairua (spirituality) and whānaungatanga (connectedness), and connected to the environment. Their world view informs a collective way of functioning, driven by associated responsibilities and obligations to each other. This contrasts markedly with a Western biomedical world view that dominates how most health services are structured and delivered. A biomedical approach tends to focus more on disease or illness, problems and individuals.

Contemporary Māori are diverse, ranging from those who have had 'traditional' Māori upbringings to those who know they are Māori but have lost their cultural and whakapapa connections (Ihimaera, 1998; Webber, 2008). Nonetheless, for many, whānau (extended family) remains the fabric of Māori society. Traditional whakapapa whānau are a 'family group' defined by common ancestors, comprising three generations who occupy a common set of building, and manage as a social and economic unit (Mead, 2003; Metge, 1995). However, for many Māori who live in urban environments, whānau comprises different forms, such as a nuclear family structure or whānau with Māori who are not necessarily related by whakapapa. Metge (1995) describes two key whānau forms:

1 whakapapa whānau whereby members are able to link their geneaolgy to a common ancestor; or
2 kaupapa whānau which comprises of members who come together for a common purpose and who receive similar benefits as those in a whakapapa whānau (such as support).

Whānau are guided by a number of values that contribute to a strong sense of collective responsibility (see Table 16.1) and are involved in:

- providing support and encouragement;
- caring and raising their members' children;
- caring and managing their property including taonga (treasures) like mātauranga (knowledge) and whakapapa;

TABLE 16.1 *Whānau values that guide members' functioning and interaction*

VALUE	DEFINITION	INFLUENCE ON WHĀNAU
Aroha	Affection, compassion, empathy, charity, love	An unconditional disposition grounded in generosity and putting others first.
Whānaungatanga	Relationships, kinship, family connections	Individuals' family connections which reinforces their responsibilities to other relatives.
Taha wairua, taha tinana	Spiritual and physical dimensions of a people	The imperative that the spiritual dimension is necessary to balance and is woven together with the physical dimension to make people complete.
Tapu and noa	Prohibited, restricted or sacred; free from tapu, respectively	Guides to keep people safe and well by making clear what has prohibitions or restrictions imposed or is sacred, and what can be freely engaged with.
Ora	To be alive, safe, well, healthy	Refers to being alive and well in a holistic sense, that is, body, mind and spirit.
Tika, tikangā, pono	Doing things the right way and being true	This is observing the appropriate moral, spiritual and social ways of doing things, and being open and honest.
Mana	Authority, power, status	Delegated spiritual power and authority that gives a person their whānau status, which can be affected by the actions of others or by members of the whānau.
Mahi-a-ngākau	Work done from, or laid upon, the heart	Prescribes a duty to support and care for one another and to protect against physical or spiritual attack, to work together for a common good.
Utu	Principle of reciprocity	Anything that is received must be appropriately returned, at some time in the future, and is essential for managing relationships between members of a whānau, as well as those outside the whānau.
Kotahitanga	Unity or sense of togetherness	Collective responsibility for each other and acting in ways that minimises or controls harm.

Source: Metge (1995)

- organising hui (gatherings) for important events (such as tangihanga (the days leading up to a funeral), unveiling of gravestones and celebrations);
- dealing with their problems and conflicts (Metge, 1995).

Collective responsibility refers to the inherent obligation that whānau members have to one another as individuals and as a whole. Therefore, whānau often function as a whole, rather than as individuals. This is often observed when a member becomes unwell in hospital and most whānau members want to tautoko (support) and manaaki (care for) the patient. This sense of collective responsibility is something that challenges many health professionals and health services. It is important to remember that whānau ngatanga is the value that binds whānau members (close and distant) in kinship, responsibility and obligation, over the needs of individual members (Patterson, 1992).

The need for whānau-focused health services

Inequities in health care for Māori are evident in relation to morbidity, mortality and use of health services. Many Māori (41%) live in the most deprived neighbourhoods (New Zealand Deprivation Index deciles 9–10, where 1=least deprivation and 10=most deprivation) compared to 15 per cent of non-Māori (Ministry of Health, 2010a). Māori also have poorer health literacy compared to other groups (Ministry of Health, 2010b). One in three Māori live with a disability (Statistics New Zealand, 2014). These all have detrimental effects on their ability to access the necessary determinants for health. Evidence of this is in the number of preventable and avoidable hospital admissions, and the mortality rates for conditions that could have been prevented or treated in the primary care setting (Ministry of Health, 2010a). Māori have a 16 per cent higher chance of an unplanned hospital readmission or death following hospitalisation (Rumball-Smith & Hider, 2013). Major causes of death include ischaemic heart disease, lung cancer, diabetes, chronic obstructive pulmonary disease, cerebrovascular disease and suicide. In 2013 the statistics for Māori death rates indicated that they lived younger than non-Māori by 7.4 years for men and 7.2 years for women (Statistics New Zealand, 2013a). Essentially, Māori die of diseases of older age before they reach this older age. In 2013 only 4.1 per cent of Māori lived beyond the age of 65 years, compared with 14.3 per cent of non-Māori (Statistics New Zealand, 2013b). In addition, Māori are also over-represented in social issues that negatively impact health such as family violence, child abuse and neglect, alcohol and drug misuse, and problem gambling.

The 2012 the New Zealand Health Survey indicated that Māori were more likely to have unmet health needs when they accessed health services (Ministry of Health, 2012). Māori accessing hospital services were more likey to experience higher adverse events rates and shorter lengths of stay (Davis et al., 2006; Rumball-Smith & Hider, 2013), and to report discrimination and racism when they used health services (Harris et al., 2012). Reid and Robson (2007) classify racism in three ways: interpersonal, institutional and personally mediated. These forms of racism result in disparities in accessing determinants of health, health care and the quality of care received.

FOR REFLECTION What are the historical, contemporary socio-economic and political contexts that impact Māori health and well-being?

Health is a human right afforded to all people. Yet, despite having multiple rights to optimal health, Māori suffer persistent inequities in health status, health outcomes and in accessing health services. Any inequities in health care are unjust and unfair. 'Equity', an ethical principle based on human rights, is about everyone having fair and just treatment. However, it should not be confused with 'equality'. Equity is about everyone having what is right for them, whereas equality relates to everyone having the same interventions or outcomes (Braveman & Gruskin, 2003). Therefore, equitable health care results in different approaches to achieve the same outcomes that others experience. Māori have multiple rights to optimal health and well-being:

- as tangata whenua under the Treaty;
- as indigenous peoples under the United Nations' *Declaration on the Rights of Indigenous Peoples* (United Nations, 2008);
- in the preamble of the United Nations' *Convention on the Rights of Persons with Disabilities* (United Nations, 2006)
- afforded under the Health and Disabilities Commissioners Act (1994) and the New Zealand Public Health and Disabilities Act (2000).

When exploring the notions of unjust inequalities, Powers and Faden (2006) claim that achieving social justice requires us to be mindful of the barriers to achieving well-being.

FOR REFLECTION What are similarities and differences in health services for Māori in your local area offered by:
> District Health Boards;
> Primary Health Organisations;
> whānau ora collectives and Māori health service providers?

Evidence exists that, prior to colonisation, Māori were fit and healthy, although today the picture differs (Kingi, 2007). That Māori have gone from a fit and healthy people, to experience the worst overall health status of those living in Aotearoa is testament to a complex history. Colonisation, and its subsequent effects, experienced by many iwi persists across generations and is compounded by poverty, discrimination and racism, and ongoing socio-economic and health inequities (Reid & Robson, 2007). Well and healthy whānau are important for the future of Māori (and Aotearoa), and for developing young people with secure attachments and strong bonds with whānau members.

Whānau ora

Whānau ora is a goal of He Korowai Oranga, the Māori Health Strategy, and the focus of health and social policy (King & Turia, 2002). The government's vision has been extended to healthy futures (pae ora) for Māori, which involves having healthy whānau (whānau ora), individuals (mauri ora) and environments (wai ora) (Ministry of Health, 2014). The pathways to achieve pae ora include supporting whānau development, Māori participation in the health and disability sector, effective service delivery and cross-sector collaboration.

Whānau ora focuses on whānau as a whole rather than on its individual members, and draws on an interagency approach to build the capacity of whānau and families living in New Zealand. For most Māori, whānau ora is not a new concept – it is a traditional holistic approach to health and well-being.

Whānau ora involves whānau identifying their health and social needs in addition to the strengths that exist within the whānau as a whole. In this way they can then establish strategies to develop necessary knowledge and skills to be able to manage their health and well-being together. This contrasts with current health service delivery approaches that attend to individuals and their problems (Te Puni Kōkiri, 2011). This means that, rather than being passive recipients of health services, whānau, hapū and iwi all have active roles in achieving their aspirations for whānau health and well-being based on their particular goals and needs (Durie et al., 2010). For many whānau, they may need the help of someone to guide them in identifying their needs and strategies.

Whānau ora, therefore, requires a different way of thinking about health service delivery for Māori, particularly the way in which health professionals practise. Rather than solely focusing on the diseases, problems and deficits that individual Māori may have about their health, health professionals need to reframe the way that they provide health services. Instead, the focus needs to:

- be on wellness and health, in ways that acknowledges the diversity within and between whānau;
- be based on what is important to whānau;
- build on the strengths of its individual members and the whānau as a collective.

What are the values, health beliefs and practices that are delivered by:
> general health services;
> Māori health services?
How may they influence the development of your practice?

Strategies for Māori- and whānau-centred practice

Māori and their whānau should remain the central focus of health professionals' activities, involving them in planning and decision-making activities, and when deciding on which services are needed to achieve their goals. Paternalistic 'we know best' attitudes are alienating, positioning Māori and their whānau as passive players in their healthcare experiences. It ignores the notion that often the answers to improving their health often lie within the whānau and community. But we need to listen and be responsive.

In what ways can a whānau-centred focus be more beneficial for Māori using health services?

The concepts of social justice (fairness), equity (different approaches to achieve equal outcomes) and Māori rights should underpin whānau-centred practice. Reframing practice, so that it is whānau-centred and identifies both the individual and the collective whānau members, ensures that whānau are able to identify and meet their own needs. Therefore, attention can focus on building knowledge, skills and capacities so that whānau can develop strategies to better meet their needs and promote healthy lifestyles. Health professionals should put aside their role to direct and control health service delivery outside of acute and potentially life-threatening or crisis situations. Māori- and whānau-centred practice is about facilitating the necessary contexts so that whānau can be empowered and their sense of agency strengthened. The following are a selection of strategies to assist in this endeavour.

Strategy 1: the Treaty-informed practice

The principles of partnership, participation and protection are legislated under the New Zealand Public Health and Disability Act (2000) to ensure compliance with the Treaty. They have also been identified as a framework that health professionals can use to implement the Treaty into their practice (King & Turia, 2002). 'Partnership' involves working with Māori and whānau by establishing relationships. In this case, the health professionals acts as a Treaty partner. Genuine efforts to work with Māori and whānau means mutually agreed goals and outcomes can be realised. Health decisions that do not involve Māori and whānau risk being inappropriate and/or unacceptable, and can leave them feeling that their needs have not been met.

Māori and whānau 'participation' is a key ingredient of any healthy partnership. For any decision to be useful and of value, Māori and whānau must be involved – they are 'experts' about their life circumstances. When involved in assessment, planning and intervention activities, they can indicate whether suggested interventions are realistic and feasible. Participation recognises the rights of Māori to equitable access and delivery of health services. So often Māori are not involved in planning activities and their life circumstances are not recognised – they are often labelled 'non-compliant' when treatment or intervention decisions about them are not undertaken.

'Protection' of health, and cultural beliefs and practices is vital for Māori and whānau to feel safe and spiritually well. Health is considered a taonga (treasure). Therefore, protection involves responding to Māori's and whānau's cultural needs and facilitating their access to, and use of, services that have frameworks for practice based on Māori philosophy, cultural values and tikanga.

Strategy 2: adopt culturally responsive practice

Contemporary Māori are diverse in terms of whānau, hapā and iwi, as well as in their different experiences of colonisation, capitalism, urbanisation and technological developments. Health professionals encounter Māori and their whānau, who range from those steeped in traditional cultural values and beliefs, are culturally well connected and speak te reo Māori (Māori language), to those who declare Māori ancestry but are culturally disconnected. Therefore, recognising these differences is crucial for tailoring their health experiences so that they are reflective of their beliefs and practices.

Culturally responsive practice requires culturally competent health professionals so that Māori and their whānau feel culturally safe, that is, their cultural needs have been respected and included in their healthcare experiences. Regulated health professionals in Aotearoa are required to demonstrate culturally competent practice under the Health Practitioners Competency Assurance

Act (2003). Cultural competence is defined in various ways. Wilson defines it as:

> ...the capability of ... [health practitioners] ... to articulate and demonstrate culturally appropriate and acceptable health services where clients feel culturally safe, [that involves a health practitioners'] ... reflexivity, knowledge, and skills, and an ability to work meaningfully with clients to meet their unique health and cultural needs ... (2008, p. 185)

Culturally responsive practice involves working with Māori and their whānau. Knowedge, action and integration (KAI) is a useful way of considering what is involved in culturally responsive care. KAI builds on cultural safety (that is, Māori and whānau experiences of being culturally safe) and focuses on the practice of health practitioners. KAI has three components:

1 **Knowledge:** understanding personal cultural values, beliefs, practices, assumptions, biases and stereotypes that are held about Māori and their whānau, and the subsequent power that these differentials may have on a health professional's practice. This also involves identifying the influence that personal values and beliefs have on professional expectations. It is important to have a critical analysis of the diverse realities of contemporary Māori and whānau as well as the historical, socio-economic and political influences shaping their health and well-being. Although there are cultural values that are recognised across hapū and iwi (see Table 16.1), it is impossible to fully 'know' Māori people's culture and its nuances.

2 **Actions:** working with Māori and whānau requires respecting them by showing genuine, non-judgemental attitudes and recognising their needs. Health professionals should be aware of Māori rights, as indigenous peoples, and reflect these in their actions. This helps avoid cultural imposition by recognising important but diverse cultural needs of each Māori and their whānau. Recognising the potential for conflicts in values, beliefs and practices, which may disrupt working effectively with Māori and their whānau, is vital. For instance, when 'Māori options' are not seen as important, it may be decided not to become familiar with the Māori- or whānau-centred services available within the community.

3 **Integration:** this is grounded in the notion that some cultural practices are important for Māori and their whānau so that they feel culturally safe and for their spiritual well-being, for example, karakia (prayer) before a procedure. Integration involves talking to each Māori and their whānau about their cultural needs or what is important for them, and including these into

their intervention plans. It is helpful to understand that whakamā (a Māori concept of shame, shyness or embarrassment) may prevent Māori and their whānau from accessing Māori services because whānau nga (relatives) work there, or cause inappropriate and/or uncomfortable environments or situations that go unrecognised by health professionals.

What changes do you need to make when working with Māori and their whānau to optimise your cultural responsiveness?

Strategy 3: engage in collaboration

Collaboration is crucial for working with communities and importantly for whānau with whom health services are offered. In addition, collaboration with interdisciplinary colleagues, whether they are community health workers or other health professionals, is essential to support whānau to achieve the outcomes they want. It is imperative for everyone to act collaboratively to achieve a positive outcome.

Principles underpinning collaborative relationships and activities include:

- having commitment;
- working together;
- having common goals;
- recognising collaboration is a journey.

Importantly, collaboration is a responsibility to work with others with a commitment to achieving the shared goal(s).

Strategy 4: know the community

Knowing the community is helpful for health professionals working with Māori and their whānau. This involves getting to know key people within relevant health and social services, including Māori health professionals. 'Knowledge is power' and the benefit of getting to know the community is twofold. It will empower the health professionals and benefit the Māori and their whānau by referring them to appropriate services.

When Māori health professionals, such as community health workers, have been identified, it is helpful to arrange a time to meet with key people. Having a Māori elder (kaumātua or kuia) attend the meeting helps ensure that tikanga is observed. District Health Boards have Māori health units, that offer guidance

about how to get the support of a kaumātua. This service is not free. Health professionals may be expected to sing a waiata (song) to support the mihi (greeting)
given by the kaumātua. A small mihi, in either English or Māori, gives details
about who a person is, where they are from and demonstrates respect for the
hosts. A hongi (pressing of noses) and ruru (shaking of hands) usually occurs at
the end of the mihi, prior to sharing kai (food). Full details on Māori protocols
can be found in Tauroa and Tauroa (1990).

Following the formalities, the hosts will be ready to hear what the health
professional has to say. The following list suggests what health practitioners
should do when meeting Māori hosts:

- Introduce yourself, the service you work for, and identify the group of
  people you work with.
- Clearly identify what service(s) are provided by your health service.
- Identify the key people you should liaise with at the Māori health service
  you are visiting.
- Discuss the Māori health service's preferred mode of referral to the service.
- Negotiate how your service can work with the Māori health service to ben-
  efit Māori and whānau.

FOR
REFLECTION

> What do you know about Māori health services that exist within your local
> area?
> What do you need to do to compile a directory of Māori health services to
> assist you working with Māori and their whānau?

It is useful to remember that the main focus of Māori health services is to
support the health needs of Māori and their whānau, therefore, such meet-
ings can clarify mutual expectations and avoid any possible misunderstandings. This information can then be documented and can be readily accessible
when Māori and whānau require additional support from the Māori health
services.

Strategy 5: build on strengths and existing health-promoting behaviours

Often health professionals centre on 'disease' or 'illness' processes, negative
assumptions and/or deficit explanations when working with Māori and their

whānau. It is easy to identify what is wrong or missing. What needs to be captured is the health-promoting activities and strengths that individuals, whānau or communities already use and can be built upon. This not only values Māori clients and their whānau but reinforces the positive health practices that are already being undertaken.

Supporting health-promoting activities does not mean that Māori and whānau need to change their 'culture' in any way – they may just have to think differently about how they do things. However, it challenges health professionals to think differently about the services they provide and to acknowledge the alternative ways that positive health outcomes can be achieved.

Te Arawa Whānau Ora Collective

Practice example 1

The Te Arawa Whānau Ora comprises six kaupapa Māori providers with common whakapapa connections, and established community networks with whānau, hapū, iwi and marae. It offers a whānau-centred service based on the values, kawa and tikanga of Te Arawa, that is, manaaki, awhina, aroha, tautoko and tiaki. The whānau-centred approach used by Te Arawa Whānau Ora Collective uses te pā harakeke (the flax bush) which is used to illustrate the interconnections that exist within members of the whānau and highlights the importance of everyone's roles. The harakeke bush (see Te Arawa Whānau Ora, 2014) describes whānau, with the very inner shoots representing mokopuna (grandchildren) or tāmariki (children), who are the future, and the surrounding inner leaves representing rangatahi (young people), matua (parents) and kokeke (grandparents), while the wider whānau and ancestors are represented by the outermost leaves. Whānau members need to work together to provide the necessary love and support, especially to those growing, for the whānau to become strong and resilient.

Te Arawa Whānau Ora believe whānau are integral to identifying and achieving their intergenerational goals and aspirations (Te Arawa Whānau Ora, 2014), and, to this end, can manage themselves and take responsibility for their own development. Therefore, whānau ora focuses on what is important for each whānau, and builds on the strengths they already possess as individuals and as a collective, and what they already do well so that they are actively involved in setting their health and social goals.

Whānau ora is inclusive of everyone, not just Māori, according to Te Arawa Whānau Ora. It focuses on whānau using their tino rangatiratanga (autonomy), an important concept for determining their dreams and deciding how they will go about living them. In this process they can realise their potential and goals with the necessary and relevant supports, unique to their plans. Nonetheless, not all whānau are ready to embark upon such journeys because they have more important or urgent issues to address first. Whānau ora is about what is important for each whānau and, therefore, it will look different for each whānau.

Accessing a service

Hera, a 40-year-old Māori woman, is the mother of five children aged between 10 and 25 years. She has two mokopuna, and their mother Maia, who lives with her. She has a history of asthma and has recently been diagnosed with Type 2 diabetes mellitus. The general practice in her neighbourhood needs to check on Hera and monitor her diabetes, following her recent admission to the emergency department. You are responsible for working with Hera and determining her needs.

Option 1

After contacting Hera twice you sense that she is reluctant to see you, but without providing an explanation, you tell her that she has to come. You document Hera as 'non-compliant' although she eventually attends the practice one day without an appointment. You reluctantly 'squeeze' her into your day, hurriedly give her pamphlets about Type 2 diabetes and suggest that she attends support groups that run in the early evenings. Hera leaves with no further understanding of her diabetes or having the reason she came to the general practice identified.

Hera will potentially re-present to a health service with poorly managed diabetes due to you *not* taking the following actions:

1 making Hera feel welcome and not rushed because she is unsure about engaging with this health service;

2 exploring her health history, her role in her whānau, her support system and inviting her to bring whānau support for future visits;

3 determining Hera's existing knowledge about Type 2 diabetes and how it can be managed;

4 ensuring Hera has a basic understanding of Type 2 diabetes and the importance of regular health

checks, especially so that she can enjoy her mokopuna growing up;

5 involving Hera in planning based on her needs to improve her understanding of Type 2 diabetes and her ongoing care (such as retinal screening, foot care and diet).

Option 2

You recognise Hera's role in managing her diabetes, and the importance of involving her in planning her health care. You also realise the importance of understanding Hera's home life and support systems, and explain, in a genuine and non-judgemental manner, why this is important for planning her care. You enquire about Hera's existing knowledge about Type 2 diabetes, and her normal nutritional and exercise habits. In addition, you determine the health-promoting behaviours she undertakes and any strengths that could assist her. Importantly, you determine what Hera's health goals are.

Following your conversation with Hera, you have established the important role that food plays when her wider whānau gathers and that she has an important role in caring for her mokopuna when she is not working. You also find out her daughter is hapū (pregnant) and recently left an abusive relationship. Together you decide that Hera needs to know more about diabetes and its management, although she prefers to undertake this learning in a Māori environment. You are also aware of a local Māori health provider and facilitate Hera to access their diabetes support programme. You also connect Hera with the local whānau ora collective, as she has whānau-related goals that are important but are beyond the resources of the general practice, especially with supporting her daughter and mokopuna.

Demonstrating a commitment to working with Hera and being focused on her needs in a genuine, non-judgemental and relaxed approach, will facilitate establishing a more effective working relationship. While option 2 involves more time, being focused about the information that you need to gather uses time more effectively and establishes a positive relationship.

Conclusion

Health professionals have a duty to act in ways that will be of most benefit to Māori and whānau, and ensure that they receive quality, safe and effective health services. As great diversity exists amongst Māori, it is important to work with each Māori person using your service and their whānau to establish their specific needs. For Māori wanting to access Māori health services, every effort should be made to facilitate this. Being knowledgeable about the Māori health services that are available in the local community or area is beneficial. Various strategies can be used to improve Māori health outcomes to build on existing health-promoting activies and strengths that Māori and whānau possess. This requires culturally responsive practice and working collaboratively with Māori and whānau.

References

Braveman, P. & Gruskin, S. (2003). Defining equity in health. *Journal of Epidemiology and Community Health, 57*(4), 254–8. doi:10.1136/jech.57.4.254

Davis, P., Lay-Yee, R., Dyall, L., Briant, R., Sporle, A., Brunt, D. & Scott, A. (2006). Quality of hospital care for Māori patients in New Zealand: Retrospective cross-sectional assessment. *The Lancet, 367*(9526), 1920–5. doi:10.1016/s0140–6736(06)68847–8

Durie, M. (1998). *Te mana, te kawanatanga: The politics of Māori self-determination.* Auckland: Oxford University Press.

Durie, M., Cooper, R., Grennell, D., Snively, S. & Tuaine, N. (2010). *Whānau ora: Report of the Taskforce on whānau-centred Initiatives.* Wellington: Ministry of Social Development.

Harris, R., Cormack, D., Tobias, M., Yeh, L.-C., Talamaivao, N., Minster, J. & Timutimu, R. (2012). The pervasive effects of racism: Experiences of racial discrimination in New Zealand over time and associations with multiple health domains. *Social Science & Medicine, 74*(3), 408–15. doi:10.1016/j.socscimed.2011.11.004

Ihimaera, W. (ed.). (1998). *Growing up Māori*. Auckland: Tandem Press.

King, A. & Turia, T. (2002). *He korowai oranga: Māori health strategy*. Wellington: Ministry of Health. Retrieved 16 November 2014 from http://www.health.govt. nz/publication/he-korowai-oranga-maori-health-strategy

Kingi, T. K. (2007). The Treaty of Waitangi: A framework for Māori health development. *New Zealand Journal of Occupational Therapy, 54*(1), 4–10.

Mead, H. M. (2003). *Tikanga Māori: Living by Māori values*. Wellington: Huia.

Metge, J. (1995). *New growth from old: The whānau in the modern world*. Wellington: Victoria University Press.

Ministry of Health. (2010a). *Tatau kahukura: Māori health chart book 2010* (2nd edn.). Wellington: Ministry of Health.

Ministry of Health. (2010b). *Korero marama: Health literacy and Māori. Results from the 2006 adult literacy and life skills survey*. Wellington: Ministry of Health.

Ministry of Health. (2012). *The health of New Zealand Adults 2011/12: Key findings of the New Zealand Health Survey*. Retrieved 16 November 2014 from http://www. health.govt.nz/publication/health-new-zealand-adults-2011–12

Ministry of Health. (2014). *He Korowai Oranga: Māori Health Strategy 2014*. Retrieved 16 November 2014 from http://www.health.govt.nz/publication/guide-he-korowai-oranga-Māori-health-strategy

Patterson, J. (1992). *Exploring Māori values*. Melbourne: Thomson Dunmore Press.

Powers, M. & Faden, R. (2006). *Social justice: The moral foundations of public health and health policy*. New York: Oxford University Press.

Reid, P. & Robson, B. (2007). Understanding health inequities. In B. Robson & R. Harris (eds.) *Hauora: Māori health standards IV. A study of the years 2000–2005* (pp. 3–10). Wellington: Te Ropu Rangahau Hauora a Eru Pomare. Retrieved 16 November 2014 from http://www.hauora.maori.nz

Robson, B., Cormack, D. & Cram, F. (2007). Social and economic indicators. In B. Robson & R. Harris (eds.) *Hauora: Māori health standards IV. A study of the years 2000–2005* (pp. 21–32). Wellington: Te Ropu Rangahau a Eru Pomare.

Rumball-Smith, J. & Hider, P. (2013). The validity of readmission rate as a marker of the quality of hospital care, and a recommendation for its definition. *New Zealand Medical Journal, 122*(1289), 64–70.

Statistics New Zealand. (2013a). *2013 Census quick statistics about Māori*. Retrieved 16 November 2014 from http://www.stats.govt.nz

Statistics New Zealand. (2013b). *2013 Census quick statistics about national highlights*. Retrieved 16 November 2014 from http://www.stats.govt.nz

Statistics New Zealand. (2014). *Disability survey: 2013*. Retrieved 16 November 2014 from http://www.stats.govt.nz/browse_for_stats/health/disabilities/ DisabilitySurvey_HOTP2013.aspx. Tauroa, H. & Tauroa, P. (1990). Te Marae: A guide to customs and protocols. Auckland: Heinemann Reed.

Tauroa, H. & Tauroa, P. (1990). *Te Marae: A guide to customs and protocols*. Auckland: Heinemann Reed.

Te Arawa Whānau Ora. (2014). *Te pā harakeke: Whānau centred service approach*. Retrieved 16 November 2014 from http://tearawawhānau ora.org.nz/about-the-collective/he-pa-harakeke/

Te Puni Kōkiri. (2011). Whānau ora fact sheet. Retrieved 16 November 2014 from http://www.tpk.govt.nz/en/a-matou-mohiotanga/whānau-ora/

United Nations. (2006). Convention on the rights of persons with disabilities. Retrieved 16 November 2014 from http://www.un.org/disabilities/convention/conventionfull.shtml

United Nations. (2008). *Declaration on the rights of indigenous peoples*. Retrieved 16 November 2014 from http://www.un.org/esa/socdev/unpfii/documents/DRIPS_en.pdf

Webber, M. (2008). *Walking the space between: Identity and Māori/Pākehā*. Wellington: NZCER Press.

Wilson, D. (2008). The significance of a culturally appropriate health service for indigenous Māori women. *Contemp Nurse, 28*(1–2), 173–88.

Wilson, D. & Barton, P. (2012). Indigenous hospital experiences: A New Zealand case study. *Journal of Clinical Nursing, 21*(15–16), 2316–26. doi:10.1111/j.1365-2702.2011.04042.x

Acknowledgements

We would like to acknowledge Ngaroma (Mala) Grant, Chief Executive of Te Arawa Whānau Ora, for her support and feedback in preparing this chapter.

Nursing and working with disability

17

Huhana Hickey

Learning objectives

Having studied this chapter, you will be able to:

- briefly explain the background to disability identity;

- briefly describe the history of models of disabilities;

- describe whānau hauā and its difference from mainstream disabilities;

- recognise cultural issues when nursing whānau hauā and individuals with disabilities.

Key terms and concepts

- disability identity

- models of disability

- whānau hauā

Introduction

Disability identity is a difficult concept because for some it is a personal decision and for others it is political. Māori are very clear that they do not identify as disabled or as people with disabilities. Māori preference to identify from a kaupapa Māori (primarily Māori) and a whakapapa (genealogical) cultural context is nothing new – what is new for many providers of health and disability services is the insistence by Māori that they be referred to as whānau hauā[1] and not as having disabilities.

[1] Whānau hauā is the preferred term for disability for Māori. This is because Māori see themselves as a whānau member first, not as their disability. The hauā derives from hau meaning wind which impacts on the environment depending on its verocity. Hauā is increasingly identified as a term to mean someone affected by the environment within which they live; alternatively someone who is diversely unique. Māori have long struggled to identify with the term disability (Hickey, 2008).

When I began my own journey into nursing in 1979, I do not recall ever having to understand any individual culturally or identify a person as having a disability. It was not until I returned to training in 1991 that I first began learning about cultural safety in nursing. It was also the first time I heard the term 'disability' which I came to understand as a political identity. In 1993 I could not complete my nursing due to early signs of primary progressive multiple sclerosis and chronic obstructive pulmonary disease from my mother who smoked around me as a child. I left nursing to undertake university study in a social science field and later completed a PhD. In the United States, nurses with disabilities are allowed to continue to practice nursing due to the American Disabilities Act (1990), after they fought for it. In New Zealand, however, this is not necessarily the case. While there are some nurses with disabilities practising, I am personally aware of several who, due to their diagnosis, have felt that they were bullied out of the profession. However, whether they can work or not depends on their nursing environment. Since my own journey in health and disability services as a client, student and practitioner, I have found that the nursing fraternity has a lot to learn about disability, in particular, to whānau hauā and other cultural identities, who are largely ignored by both the cultural and disability communities (Hickey, 2008).

Disabilities identity: a brief introduction

In 1975, with the development of the Social Model of Disability through the Union of the Physically Impaired Against Segregation (UPIAS) (Campbell & Oliver, 1996), 'disability discourse' emerged as a label/terminology from the medical, social work and rehabilitation fields. This, in turn, has changed to 'disability identity' due to the creation of identity-based critical fields of study (including women's and queer-based studies). Disability identity is briefly discussed in this chapter to incorporate an understanding of disability, as an identity, and identity issues. Disability identity work is increasingly recognising and acknowledging the diversity that exists within our different communities. Along with this gain in knowledge, is an understanding of the complicated factors that have impacted on these different identity frameworks. The identity of indigenous people with disabilities is inextricably linked to ethnicity and gender status, and yet little research has been carried out to explore these intersectionalities and their impact on the well-being of indigenous people with disabilities. Research undertaken has been driven from a health professional's perspective and focuses on how to provide culturally appropriate services regarding the health status of indigenous peoples. Little analysis has been done from the position of identity around indigeneity and disability.

> The distinction between impairment and disability lies at the heart of the social model…impairment is defined in individual and biological terms. Disability is defined as a social creation…For social modellists, social barriers and social oppression constitute disability, and this is the area where research, analysis, campaigning and change must occur. (Shakespeare, 2006, p. 34)

Disability identity is a socially and politically constructed identity and therefore has not existed outside of models of disability. Impairment, on the other hand, has always presented as a medical diagnosis of a particular condition affecting an individual. Disability identity has evolved from the industrialisation of society. The word 'impairment' has been used to denote a common denominator for a group of people having a similar disability. The word impairment is confined to individual experiences a physical presentation of a medical condition, whereas the word 'disability' emcompasses experiences of marginalisation and discrimination. The difficulty in acknowledging the identity of disability is that, with impairment, comes the loss of identifying positively about self and having to adopt an identity which has terminologies fixed in deficit language. Disability identity is linguistically specific in its formation As a result, disability identity is complicated to define with other identities such as being Māori and living with disabilities. This is known as the identity of 'other' (Galvin, 2003). Identity, and the interaction of power relationships, can lead through language, to create that identity of 'other'. An example of this is the term 'disability' for Māori, which has negative connotations attached through the use of the term 'disability', whereas using the preferred term 'whānau hauā' has a more positive language attached to its meaning and therefore its use is more acceptable among Māori. This leads Māori to being more amenable to accepting disability issues within their community (Hickey, 2008).

The process of 'othering' is applicable to identities that fit outside the concept of what was perceived as natural and leads to the negative fears around disability identity (Foucault, 1988; Hughes, 2000). Brown (2002, p. 41) states that:

> For the development of disability culture, history of disabled people has an important role to play. History occupies a significant place in the formation of group identity. However, until recently, history of disabled people has been ignored.

Brown argues that disability identity history has been ignored except through the medical aspects of disability, where attention is given to disability from an objectification of the individual's identity based on medical frameworks (Brown, 2002). As other aspects of disability identity, such as feminism and disability, have developed, so has the understanding of disability as an identity (Corker & Shakespeare, 2002; Foucault, 1988; Garland-Thompson, 2002; Morris, 1991; 1993; Oliver, 1996). For those who are interested in reading further, there are a range of resources available to learn more about disability as an identity.

Because diversity of understanding impairment exists within different cultural communities, some indigenous people believe that some impairments have a social or spiritual component which affects well-being but does not derive from a medical or physiological condition. Some indigenous communities, such as the African Kigali people, sadly do not encourage tribal members with disabilities to participate, hence the exclusion and isolation that often occurs for some indigenous people with disabilities. This is often due to superstitions or ignorance around disability that are centuries old. Indigenous communities, who experienced colonisation, have been exposed to missionaries, whose attitudes towards disability have influenced their thinking. The diversity of experiences within indigenous communities towards disability, therefore, is similar to the diversity of experiences within non-indigenous communities.

Hemi

Practice example 1

Hemi, an 18-year-old male, lives in South Auckland. He has been living with his mother and five younger siblings in a Housing New Zealand home. Hemi has never worked, he has just left high school and was considering further study in sports and recreation, as his main interest is rugby. His father hasn't been in his life since he was five years old. Hemi is in the Otara Spinal Unit, as he has sustained a major spinal injury in a car accident leaving him a quadriplegic with minimal mobility. Hemi is Māori and Samoan. He is due for release back home soon. You are responsible for working with Hemi and ascertaining his requirements.

Meeting 1
After meeting with Hemi, you have determined him to be scared and angry, with a sense of losing hope around him. He does not want to go back home and feels that his mother is taking over his life. He is reluctant to work with you and so you have, in your report, labelled him as non-compliant and a risk to himself and his whānau.

Meeting 2
You arrange to meet with him again, with some suggestions for him to help him address his fears. You leave him with some information about support groups and suggest that he talks with some of the other residents at the

spinal unit. You also suggest a meeting with him and his mother to begin the journey of getting him home. He shrugs his shoulders but agrees to a meeting.

Meeting 3

Hemi appears ready to talk to you. He has been speaking to other residents of the spinal unit. He is keen to sort some things out so that he can get out of the unit.

FOR REFLECTION

> What do you propose to do given that there is a need for some changes at home, or where he chooses to live, to enable him to go home?
> Who would you involve in his rehabilitation plan?
> How would you bring the whānau together for a meeting and who would be at that meeting?
> What community networks would be useful for him to know about and what professional services will he need for his long-term care?

Practice example continued

As you are the primary careworker, it is your job to ensure that he is fully prepared for his release from the spinal unit to the community. It is your job to know what is needed to assist him to be independent.

FOR REFLECTION

How is disability identity constructed and is that construction problematic for other groups with disability?

Māori/indigenous disability identity

In New Zealand, indigenous people with disabilities also have the added issue of facing greater discrimination due, in part, to the lack of culturally appropriate services and the social, economic placement of disability within society. Added to this is the overall lack of appropriate support from the government and its agencies for all indigenous peoples. Until indigenous people receive appropriate support, indigenous people with disabilities cannot expect to see improvements in their own status (Durst & Bluechardt, 2001).

The often used term 'oppression' is not appropriate in the context of indigenous peoples with disability as it holds a negative assumption that may not always be the case. 'Triple jeopardy', which also has an implication of negativity, has a slightly different emphasis. 'Jeopardy' implies that, while oppression may occur, all three identities have a historical foundation of marginalisation.

Therefore, even if not oppressed by society, the identities alone have a component of marginalisation. With more than two marginalised identities already attached to the individual, if a third marginalised identity is added to the existing ones, then there is a triple impact of marginalisation which is very difficult for the individual to avoid. This triple impact is identified as 'triple jeopardy' (Durst & Bluechardt, 2001). Ghai (2003, p. 80), in describing colonisation and disability, states that:

> The colonised loses its entity as a subject in its own right and remains only what the coloniser is not. It is thus an erasure both out of history and all significant aspects of development.

Despite society believing that indigenous people with disabilities have a disability, there may be a difference in perception between the health and disability professionals, and indigenous peoples, who may not see themselves as having a disability (Gething, 1995). When Gething explored what constituted a personal definition of disability, it was found that there was a lack of clear statistical significance of what constitutes a disability between the professionals and the Aboriginal people themselves. Obvious impairments, such as amputations or severe physical impairments, are easily defined as a disability; it is the hidden impairments such as intellectual/learning or psychosocial which are often not seen as a disability by indigenous people generally. Many of the disabilities that affect us later in life are considered to be a normal aspect of the life cycle and are therefore not singled out or isolated as belonging to the disability identity. 'Disability is rarely seen as a separate issue, but is seen as part of problems which are widespread and a part of the life cycle' (Gething, 1995).

Therefore, the term 'disability' does not exist for some cultural groups and thus they do not consider attributing this identity. If, for example, deaf Māori wish to construct themselves not as a disability identity but as Māori who identify within the deaf cultural framework, then it is their right to do so. Furthermore, what could be viewed as a disability today differs between the different cultural and tribal beliefs of indigenous peoples. What the dominant Western ideology may define as a disability may not be the same for different indigenous peoples (Coleridge, 1993).

The exclusion for Māori with disabilities is the invisibility of identity, leading to the lack of consideration and often financial resources where access is an issue. For example, in June 2006, the Ministry of Health held hui in Auckland, which was one of only three hui held countrywide. This therefore excluded many out-of-town Māori with disabilities who did not have the resources to attend.

Another example, highlighting some concerns of whānau hauā, was the use of service dogs, such as guide dogs, and their ability to go onto marae without opposition from the mana whenua of that marae. The Ngāti Kāpō advocacy group for Māori who are blind raised the issue of their guide dogs on marae at these hui, and objections were raised by the members of the local marae to having these dogs within the buildings. This is a common problem for Ngāti Kāpō members and now others with service dogs, who assert their right to independence by having their guide dogs with them when they attend any hui.

Some of the older marae have not been modernised or updated with ramps or sensory aids to assist anyone who has an impairment. Some, but not all, of the newer marae have addressed this with accessible toilets and bathroom areas, and ramps instead of steps into the whare.

Full participation in society means having a full and meaningful involvement with economic, social and leisure activities. Unfortunately, for many indigenous people, this is denied due to economic factors. Indigenous people with disabilities face further marginalisation because it is highly unlikely that they will be employed or will be able to access their health and equipment needs, in order to be able to participate in employment. Therefore, they face the double jeopardy of both identities.

Statistics

In relation to statistics for Māori with disabilities, the 2013 census statistics show that, while approximately one in four New Zealanders have some form of disability (25%), more than one in three (32%) Māori identify as whānau hauā (Statistics New Zealand, 2014). More strikingly, just under half of whānau hauā are under the age of 25 years (Statistics New Zealand, 2014). The median age for disability for Māori is 40 years whereas for European it is 57 years. Māori children under the age of 15 had a disability rate of 15 per cent, compared with nine per cent for non-Māori children (Statistics New Zealand, 2014).

The Māori disability rate reflects four main impairment types: psychological/psychiatric impairments; difficulty with learning; difficulty with speaking; and intellectual disability. However, Statistics New Zealand (2014) showed that Māori also had slightly higher rates of vision impairment and slightly lower rates of mobility impairment than non-Māori. There was no difference between disability rates for Māori men (32%) and Māori women (31%), but Māori boys experienced disability at a higher rate than Māori girls (19% and 10%, respectively). Statistics New Zealand (2014) showed that whānau hauā were highly likely to be unemployed (48%) compared to non-Māori, and over 60 per cent lived on $15 000 or less. It would appear that whānau hauā experience inequalities and inequities when accessing and using services at a greater rate than others living in New Zealand, despite having the right to equal outcomes affirmed under Article 3 of the Treaty of Waitangi (Derret et al., 2011; Harwood, 2010).

Whānau hauā have been disporportionately represented in the disability and deprivation statistics (Statistics New Zealand, 2014). Whānau hauā have less productivity and less quality of life than non-Māori directly caused by the inequitable experiences of disability. Only 16 per cent of whānau hauā access Ministry of Health-funded disability support services (The Centre, 2014). Whānau hauā comprise 37.8 per cent under the age of 15 years and 49 per cent under the age of 25 years. Fifty-one per cent of whānau hauā have a learning/intellectual disability and 32.2 per cent have a physical disability. Notably, almost one in four (23%) of whānau hauā have a signifcant or very high health need (The Centre, 2014).

Mere

Practice example 2

Mere is a 52-year-old woman, she is in a relationship and has four children aged five to 21. She has one mokopuna, who she and her partner have taken responsibility for, because her daughter is unable to care for her. Mere has been told that she has a form of muscular dystrophy and has been released from hospital to her home in a wheelchair. Mere is unable to get to her general practice. You have been given responsibility to follow her up to ascertain her needs.

Meeting 1
You find Mere is alone with her tamariki and mokopuna, her partner has left and her daughter, the mother of the mokopuna, has returned home to help care for her mother. Mere has bed sores and she is struggling to use the wheelchair, as it was not set up for her specific body needs. The house has no ramp and while she is in a Housing New Zealand home, Mere has struggled to pay the rent and is being threatened with eviction. As Mere is housebound, she has been unable to get to the bank or to any of the services that she needs. Mere appears depressed and withdrawn. She has no service overseeing her needs.

> What is Mere's immediate need that you must attend to?
> What services need to work with Mere and her whānau?
> What Māori services would be useful for Mere and her whānau?

FOR REFLECTION

Practice example continued

You arrange, in agreement with Mere, a hui of service providers for Mere to address short-term and long-term support for her and her whānau. What are the things you need to consider to make sure that Mere has full support during the hui and after?

Consider the identity of disability and the difficulties for many indigenous peoples to embrace the term. Given that New Zealand has been colonised for over 175 years, why do you believe whānau hauā struggle to improve their personal circumstances and remain dominant in the negative statistics?

Models of disability

The approach to disability which I recommend is based on the premise that disability is always an interaction between individual and structural factors. Rather than getting fixated on defining disability either as a deficit or a structural disadvantage, a holistic understanding is required. The experience of people with disabilities results from the relationship intrinsic to them, and extrinsic factors arising from the wider context in which they find themselves. Among the intrinsic factors are issues such as: the nature and severity of impairment, own attitudes to impairment, personal qualities and abilities, and personality. Among the contextual factors are: the attitudes and reactions of others, the extent to which the environment is enabling or disabling, and wider cultural, social and economic issues relevant to disability in society (Shakespeare, 2006).

There are nine models that reflect changes in society's attitudes about disability (Table 17.1). These models are well researched; however, while New Zealand is promoting the social model of disability, service providers such as the disability support link, which allocates carer support hours to community-based disability services, still utilise the medical/rehabilitation/professional models when providing services to clients with disabilities, and the rights-based model when advocating for individuals with disabilities, not necessarily addressing the issues of collective identities such as indigenous persons with disabilities.

TABLE 17.1 *The nine disability models*

MODEL	DEFINITIONS
Tragic/pity/charity	Victims are seen as tragic.
	People are not seen as individuals with value but something to shun, pity and be afraid of. (Shakespeare, Mercer & Barnes, 1999)
	For example, fundraising advertising for disability organisations, such as where a child with a disability is used to induce people to give to the charity.
Religious/moral	Disability is viewed as a punishment or infliction on the individual and/or family from an external force.
	Sometimes the disability inflicts a lower status on the whole family affecting their stand in their community. The disability is inevitably seen as the result of a sin or indiscretion caused by the individual and their family, hence the rationale for punishing, isolating or even excluding the individual and their family from their community. (Clapton & Fitzgerald, 1997)
	Psychosocial conditions may be seen as being the result of 'evil spirits'.
Medical	Disability is a result of an individual's physical or mental limitations.
	The disability is largely unconnected to the social or geographical environments. (Clapton & Fitzgerald, 1997; Campbell & Oliver, 1996)
	It is sometimes referred to as the biological–inferiority or functional–limitation model.
Expert/professional	An arm of the medical model, sees the impairment as being the identifying factor with the provider being the fixer of the situation and the fixee being passive and accepting of the paternalism imposed on them. (Clapton & Fitzerald, 1997)
Rehabilitation	Another arm of the medical model, sees the disability as a deficiency with the only recourse of fixing the problem with the engagement of a professional. (Clapton & Fitzgerald, 1997; Campbell & Oliver, 1996)
Economic	Bases itself on the level of or lack of productivity by people with disabilities in the workforce.
	This is primarily policy framed around economic development and the role, or lack of, of people with disabilities. (Charlton, 2000)
Social	Identifies disability as a consequence of environmental, societal and attitudinal factors. (Campbell & Oliver, 1996; Shakespeare, 1998; Shakespeare, Mercer & Barnes, 1999; UPIAS, 1976)
Customer/empowering	This is the opposite of the professional/expert model with the professional working alongside the client and not making the decisions for the client. (Oliver, 1996; Corker & Shakespeare, 2002)
Rights-based	Conceptualises disability as a socio-political construct within a rights-based discourse and based on the social model of disability. The focus shifts from dependence to independence and bases itself within a political civil rights framework challenging ableism, racism and sexism. (Breslin & Lee, 2002; Lawson & Gooding, 2005; Shakespeare, 1998; Shakespeare, Mercer & Barnes, 1999)

There is no disability model for Māori disability identity. There are, however, several Māori health and well-being models (Nikora et al., 2004). Te Whare Tapa Whā model, designed and outlined by Professor Mason Durie, is the most commonly cited model in Māori health and development policies. At a health hui in Palmerston North in 1982, Durie presented the Whare Tapa Whā model as a four-part framework resembling the four walls of a whare (house). This analogy was made to ensure strength and symmetry, thereby giving balance in the well-being of the individual and the community. The four dimensions are:

- taha wairua (the spiritual side);
- taha hinengaro (thoughts and feelings);
- taha tinana (the physical side);
- taha whānau (family) (Durie, 1994, p. 70).

The Whare Tapa Whā model is referred to in other chapters in this book, and therefore I won't go into it here, other than to outline they are as important when considering issues around disability as they are to health.

FOR REFLECTION

Given that whānau hauā do not have a specific disability model or a specific Māori model of disability, is it possible to combine models to provide an effective culturally based service for a whānau hauā?

The nurse's role when working with clients with disabilities

When working with people with disabilities/whānau hauā, it is important to remember that these individuals, regardless of their ethnic identity, are whānau members first. If they cannot articulate their needs, then it is highly likely that their whānau will have a good understanding of their condition and their needs. A good deal of common sense is needed for disability needs in care. As well as good communication.asking appropriate questions helps to develop good relationships. Whānau hauā members may well need to liaise with cultural advisors and may wish to have their whānau stay with them as they know them better than any nursing staff.

When going into people's home environments, health professionals must remember not to judge them, as many struggle within and below the poverty line. If spending time with them, they should take something to eat, take off their shoes at the door and be guided by their hosts. Essentially, the considerations around culture are the same as with anyone else in need of health services. The only difference is the issue of disability and what that means to the individual and their whānau from their cultural view point.

Consider the client's needs when engaging with them. How would you address the concerns of the whānau and the individual with disabilities if there is a conflict?

FOR REFLECTION

Conclusion

Every disability is unique. Health professionals must remember to treat people individually rather than assume that all people with the same condition are exactly alike. This is simplistic and potentially unsafe. Every person has a unique identity – age, gender and ethnicity are all parts of this. Where, how and when they acquired their impairment all play an additionally unique part in their outlook together with what support can be available to them. Health professionals need to be aware of the complexities of disability identity and not assume that it is homogenous in nature. Rather, it is diverse in nature with layers of complexity that can only be understood through respect, understanding and treating individuals as a human being with needs that often fit outside the needs of others who can see, hear, are cognitively capable and are mobile in their everyday lives.

References

Breslin, M. L. & Lee, S. (eds). (2002). *Disability rights law and policy: International and national perspectives*. Ardsley, NY: Transnational Publishers.

Brown, S. E. (2002, Spring). What is a disability culture? *Disability Studies Quarterly, 22*(2), 34–50.

Campbell, J. & Oliver, M. (1996). *Disability politics: Understanding our past, changing our future*. London: Routledge.

Charlton, J. I. (2000). *Nothing about us without us: Disability oppression and empowerment*. Oakland: University of California Press.

Clapton J. & Fitzgerald, J. (1997, Fall). The history of disability: A history of 'otherness'. *New Renaissance magazine, 7*(1).

Coleridge, P. (1993). *Disability, liberation, and development*. Oxford: Oxfam.

Corker, M. & Shakespeare, T. (eds). (2002). *Disability/postmodernity embodying disability theory*. London: Continuum.

Derrett, S., Davie, G., Ameratunga, S., Wyeth, E., Colhoun, S., Wilson, S., Samaranayaka, A.,... & Langley, P. (2011). Prospective outcomes of injury study: Recruitment, and participant characteristics, health and disability status. *Inj Prev, 17*, 415–18. doi:10.1136/injuryprev-2011–040044

Durie, M. (1994). *Whaiora: Māori health development*. Auckland: Oxford University Press.

Durst, D. & Bluechardt, M. (2001, March). *Urban Aboriginal persons with disabilities: Double jeopardy*. Canada: University of Regina.

Foucault, M. (1988). Confinement, psychiatry, prison. In L. Kritzman (ed.) *Politics, philosophy, and culture: Interviews and other writings, 1977–1984* (pp. 178–210). New York: Routledge.

Galvin, R. (2003, Spring). The making of the disabled identity: A linguistic analysis of marginalisation. *Disability Studies Quarterly, 23*(2), 149–78.

Garland-Thompson, R. (2002). Integrating disability, transforming feminist theory. *NWSA Journal, 14*(3), 1–32.

Gething, L. (1995). A case study of Australian Aboriginal people with disabilities. *Australian Disabilities Review, 2*(1), 77–87.

Ghai, A. 2003. *(Dis)embodied form: Issues of disabled women*. New Delhi: Haranand Publications PVT Ltd.

Harwood, M. (2010). Rehabilitation and indigenous peoples: The Māori experience. *Disability and Rehabilitation, 32*(12), 972–7.

Hickey, S. J. (2008). The unmet legal social cultural needs of Māori with disabilities. Unpublished PhD, The University of Waikato, Hamilton.

Hughes, B. (2000). Medicine and the aesthetic invalidation of disabled people. *Disability and Society, 15*(4), 555–68.

Lawson, A. & Gooding, C. (eds). (2005). *Disability rights in Europe*. Oxford: Hart Publishing.

Morris, J. (1991). *Pride against prejudice: Transforming attitudes to disability*. London: The Women's Press Ltd.

Morris, J. (1993). Feminism and disability. *Feminist Review, 43*, 57–70.

Nikora, L., Karapu, R., Hickey, H. & Te Awekotuku, N. (2004). *Disabled Māori and disability support options: A report prepared for the Ministry of Health*. Hamilton: Māori & Psychology Research Unit.

Oliver, M. (1996). *Understanding disability: From theory to practice*. New York: St Martins Press.

Shakespeare. T. (2006). *Disability rights and wrongs*. London: Routledge.

Shakespeare, T. (ed.). (1998). *The disability reader: Social science perspectives*. London: Continuum.

Shakespeare, T., Mercer, G. & Barnes, C. (1999). *Exploring disability: A sociological introduction*. Cambridge: Polity Press.

Statistics New Zealand. (2014). *Disability Survey: 2013*. Wellington: New Zealand.

The Centre (2014) *Haua Mana Māori: Living unique and enriched lives*. Dunedin: University of Otago. Retrieved 20 November 2014 from http://www.health.govt.nz/

Index

Printed in the United States
by Baker & Taylor Publisher Services